Suicide –
An unnecessary death

Edited by
Danuta Wasserman, MD, PhD
Swedish National Centre for Suicide Research
and Prevention of Mental Ill-Health
Stockholm, Sweden

Martin Dunitz

In 1882, Jules Michelet wrote the following existential reflection on Vincent van Gogh's drawing Sorrow: 'Comment se fait-il qu'il y ait sur la terre une femme seule – . . .' This reflection brings to the fore the role of solitude and loneliness.

Suicide is a predominantly male phenomenon. Millions of mothers, wives, sisters and daughters are left alone in indescribable grief. Along with the male relatives, they are survivors tormented by sorrow and pain.

However, suicide is also becoming a female phenomenon. Our contemporary world, with its fascinating opportunities for development, has a shadowy side that most of us seek to avoid. An increasing number of girls and women, hurt in their loneliness and abandonment, and in their sense of exclusion from human fellowship, can no longer cope with life. In some countries, for some age groups, female suicide outnumbers male suicide.

The words of grief kill none.
Dumb silence is what kills.
Speaking, we live;
Speechless, we die.
Listen, then, to my voice –
a paltry flame that lights up
the walls of our cave.
'There is no one here,
there is nothing to fear
as long as the world exists
and the flame is lit.'

Olof Lagercrantz
(Swedish poet, born 1911)

© Martin Dunitz 2001

Front cover illustration © The New Art Gallery   Walsall, Garman Ryan Collection, UK.

Although every effort has been made to ensure that all owners of copyright material have been acknowledged in this publication, we would be glad to acknowledge in subsequent reprints or additions any omissions brought to our attention.

First published in the United Kingdom in 2001 by:
Martin Dunitz Ltd
The Livery House
7–9 Pratt Street
London NW1 0AE

Tel: +44 (0)20-7482 2202
Fax: +44 (0)20-7267 0159
E-mail: info.dunitz@tandf.co.uk
Website: http://www.dunitz.co.uk

A CIP record for this book is available from the British Library

ISBN 1-85317-822-5

Distributed in the United States by:
Blackwell Science Inc
Commerce Place, 350 Main Street
Malden MA 02148, USA
Tel: 1 800 215 1000

Distributed in Canada by:
Login Brothers Book Company
324 Salteaux Crescent
Winnipeg, Manitoba R3J 3T2
Canada
Tel: 1 204 224 4068

Distributed in Brazil by:
Ernesto Reichmann Distribuidora de Livros, Ltda
Rua Coronel Marques 335, Tatuape 03440-000
São Paulo
Brazil

Composition by Wearset, Boldon, Tyne and Wear
Printed and bound in Great Britain by Biddles Ltd, Guildford and King's Lynn

Contents

About the editor

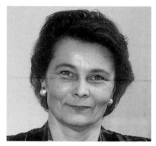

Danuta Wasserman, MD, PhD, is Professor of Psychiatry and Suicidology at the National Institute for Psychosocial Medicine/Karolinska Institute in Stockholm, Sweden and also Head of the National Swedish and Stockholm County Centre, and WHO Collaborating Centre on Suicide Research and Prevention of Mental Ill-Health. Professor Wasserman also has experience of clinical practice with depressive and suicidal patients.

Professor Wasserman studied medicine and psychology at Uppsala University. She received psychiatric training and defended her doctoral dissertation at the Karolinska Institute in Stockholm. Professor Wasserman has also completed psychoanalytical training at the Swedish Psychoanalytical Institute.

Professor Wasserman's research focuses on an interdisciplinary approach that elucidates psychodynamic, psychiatric, and genetic aspects of suicidal behaviour. The study of suicidal communication and responses of the closest family members and the care-givers, as well as psychological problems arising in patients and in the staff in the treatment process, are of particular interest to Professor Wasserman's research. An understanding of the suicidal patient's specific manner of communicating their suicidal thoughts and their psychological defence mechanisms (often misinterpreted by relatives and health-care personnel as evidence of strength and capability) are important in the treatment process.

In spite of the benefits of individual psychopharmacological management, treatment failure can often result from a suicidal patient's perceptions of and reaction to their doctors, and the doctors' and other care staff's difficulty in handling the situation. The interpersonal relationship between the suicidal patient and the doctor or the therapist, as well as between the suicidal patient and the closest significant others, are of crucial importance to the life or death of the suicidal patient.

The National Swedish and Stockholm County Centre, which Professor Wasserman founded in 1993, is active in four main areas: research and development of new suicide-preventive methods, epidemiological surveillance, information and teaching. High priority is given to projects designed to promote new suicide-preventive measures aimed at young people. The Centre's researchers collaborate in international projects.

Professor Wasserman is a member of the International Academy for Suicide Research, the International Association for Suicide Prevention, the American Academy of Suicidology, The American Foundation for Suicide Prevention, The International Psychoanalytical Association, and in various psychiatric associations. In 1993 she received the Stengel Research Award from the International Association for Suicide Prevention in recognition of her research on suicide prevention, as well as an award from the Swedish Medical Society.

About the contributors

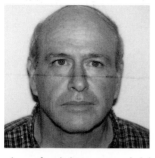

Alan Apter

Alan Apter, MD, is Professor and Chairman of the Department of Psychiatry at the Sackler School of Medicine, Tel Aviv, Israel. He is the Director of the Feinberg Child Study Center and the Department of Psychiatry at Schneider's Children's Hospital of Israel. Professor Apter's main fields of research include the genetics and neurobiology of suicide, psychological autopsies of adolescent suicide, and suicide in adolescent psychiatric patients.

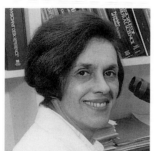

Victoria Arango

Dr Victoria Arango is an Associate Professor in the Department of Psychiatry at the New York State Psychiatric Institute at Columbia University. Dr Arango's current research focuses on the examination of monoamine systems in suicide victims and the effect of alcohol dependence on those receptor systems.

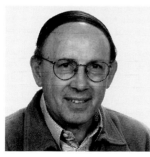

Per Bech

Per Bech, MD, is Professor of Psychiatry and Head of the Psychiatric Research Unit at the WHO Collaborating Centre, Frederiksborg General Hospital, Denmark. He was awarded the Anna Monika Prize for studies on the use of rating scales in 1983, the Duphar Antidepressant Award in 1991, and the Mölnlycke Quality of Life Award in 1997. Professor Bech's main research interests are psychometrics, depression and quality of life.

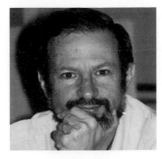

José M Bertolote

José M Bertolote, MD, is Coordinator of the Team on Management of Mental and Brain Disorders at WHO headquarters in Geneva, Switzerland, where he is responsible for SUPRE, the WHO Global Initiative on Suicide Prevention. Dr Bertolote is also Associate Professor at the Department of Psychogeriatrics at Lausanne University, Switzerland.

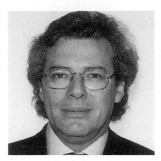

Diego De Leo

Diego De Leo, MD, is Professor of Psychiatry and Suicidology at the Griffith University, Mount Gravatt Campus, Brisbane, Australia, where he also directs the Australian Institute for Suicide Research and Prevention. Professor De Leo is the President of the International Association for Suicide Research and Prevention, and Past-President of the International Academy for Suicide Research. Professor De Leo received the 1991 Stengel Research Award.

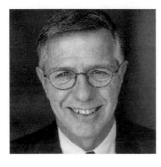

Edward J Dunne

Edward J Dunne, PhD, is a clinical psychologist in private practice in New York City. In addition he is a senior faculty member of the Ackerman Institute for the Family, where he directs the clinic for gay and lesbian families. He is the current president of the American Association of Suicidology (2000–2001), and a former chairman of its Survivor Division. He is a consultant to several survivor groups in the New York City area. Dr Dunne is the 1999 recipient of the International Association for Suicide Prevention and Crisis Intervention's Norman Farberow Award for his work with survivors.

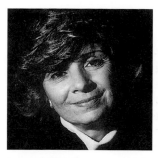

Karen Dunne-Maxim

Karen Dunne-Maxim, MS, RN, is an international expert on issues related to the survivors of suicide. She is the Coordinator for Suicide Prevention Projects at the University of Medicine and Dentistry of New Jersey – University Behavioral HealthCare at Piscataway. She has developed innovative models for responding to the special needs of families and school systems following a suicide and has been a pioneer in the effort to enlighten the public about this form of death and to eliminate the stigma often associated with it. She was the recipient of the Paloma Award from the American Foundation for Suicide Prevention in 1990, the Excellence Award from UMDNJ in 1992 and has also received the Farberow Award 1999 from the International Association of Suicide Prevention.

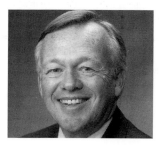

Jan Fawcett

Jan Fawcett, MD, Professor and Chairman of the Department of Psychiatry at Rush-Presbyterian-St Luke's Medical Center, is a graduate of Yale University School of Medicine. He received his psychiatric training at Langley Porter Neuropsychiatric Institute and at the University of Rochester Medical Center. Professor Fawcett's career in research began at the Clinical Center of the National Institute of Mental Health (NIMH) in Bethseda, Maryland where he became involved with research concerning the biomedical aspects of depression and suicide. In 1966 he establish a Depression Research Unit at the Illinois State Psychiatric Institute, Chicago, to study the pharmacology and biochemistry of depression as well as the prediction and prevention of suicide. Professor Fawcett was presented the Lifetime Achievement Award by American Foundation for Suicide Prevention in 2000.

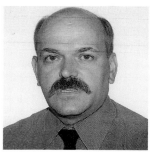

Antoon Leenaars

Antoon Leenaars, PhD, CPsych, is a psychologist in private practice in Windsor, Canada, and is a member of the Faculty at the University of Leiden, The Netherlands. He was the first Past President of the Canadian Association for Suicide Prevention (CASP), and is a past President of the American Association of Suicidology (AAS). He has published ten books and is Editor-in-Chief of Archives of (*Suicide Studies Suicide Research*). Dr Leenaars has received both CASP's Research Award and AAS's Edwin Shneidman Award.

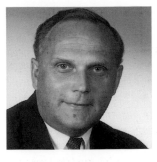

Jouko Lönnqvist

Jouko Lönnqvist, MD, is Professor and Director of the Department of Mental Health and Alcohol Research at the National Public Health Institute in Helsinki, Finland. His main research areas have been self-destructive behaviour and suicide prevention, substance abuse, psychiatric genetics and epidemiology. He has published about 200 research articles in international journals. Professor Lönnqvist received the Stengel Research Award in 1981.

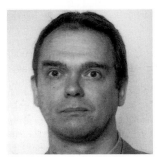

Ilkka Henrik Mäkinen

Ilkka Henrik Mäkinen, PhD, is a sociologist and currently research fellow at the University College of South Stockholm. His doctoral thesis examined suicide in European countries, and his special interests include the epidemiology and sociology of suicide, as well as attitudes, laws and the history related to this form of death.

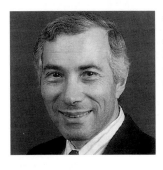

J John Mann

J John Mann, MD, is Head of the Department of Neuroscience at the New York State Psychiatric Institute and is Professor of Psychiatry and Radiology at Columbia University College of Physicians and Surgeons. Professor Mann's research employs functional brain imaging, neurochemistry, and molecular genetics to probe the causes of depression and suicide. He is Head of the NIMH-funded Clinical Research Center for the Study of Suicidal Behavior at Columbia University, the Stanley Foundation Center for the Applied Neuroscience of Bipolar Disorders, and Chairman of the Scientific Council of the American Foundation for Suicide Prevention. Professor Mann has edited nine books on suicide and psychiatric disorders.

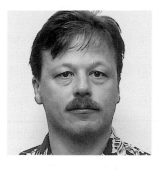

Lars Mehlum

Lars Mehlum, MD, PhD, is Professor of Psychiatry and Suicidology at the University of Oslo and founder and head of the Norwegian National Suicide Research and Prevention Centre. Dr Mehlum's research has focussed on suicidal behaviour in the young, patients with personality disorders and schizophrenia, and treatment outcome studies on suicide attempters. He is a policy adviser for suicide prevention and a board member of the International Association for Suicide Prevention, and was awarded the King's Gold Medal in 1995.

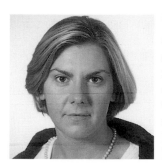

Gaia Meneghel

Gaia Meneghel, graduated in Medicine in 1996, specialised in Psychiatry and Psychotherapy in 2000 at Padua University, Italy. She currently cooperates at both clinical and research level with the WHO Collaborating Centre for Training and Research in Suicide Prevention and the Psychogeriatric Service of the Department of Psychiatry and Neurology of Padua University.

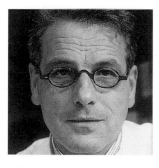

Hans-Jürgen Möller

Hans-Jürgen Möller is Professor of Psychiatry and Chairman of the Department of Psychiatry at the Ludwig-Maximilans University, Munich, Germany. His main areas of research are methodology of clinical research in psychiatry, biological psychiatry of depression, suicide and schizophrenia, clinical psychopharmacology and psychogeriatrics. He has published extensively and is chief editor of *The World Journal of Biological Psychiatry*, and is main editor, editor or member of the editorial board of several national and international psychiatric journals. He is currently president of the World Federation of Societies of Biological Psychiatry.

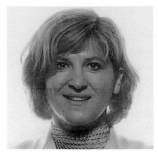

Véronique Narboni

Véronique Narboni, MD, is Guest Researcher at the Karolinska Institute in Stockholm, Sweden. She was previously involved in the creation of comprehensive educational material directed at psychiatrists in order to improve the quality of life of patients experiencing mood disorders. Dr Narboni's current area of research is the impact of educational programmes on the attitudes and behaviour of general practitioners, with particular regard to suicide prevention.

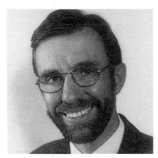

Anders Niméus

Anders Niméus, MD, is a psychiatrist and has been head of a suicide research ward since 1994 (Lund, Sweden). His main research concerns the clinical usefulness of psychiatric rating scales with special reference to scales for identifying risk for suicidal behaviour.

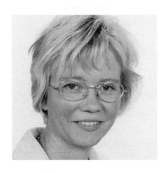

Lis Raabaek Olsen

Lis Raabaek Olsen MD works at the Psychiatric Research Unit, Frederiksborg General Hospital, Hilleröd, Denmark. Her main research areas include psychiatry, depression, distress, and the use of questionnaires.

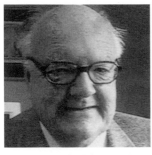

Nils Retterstøl

Nils Retterstøl, MD, is Professor Emeritus of Psychiatry, at the University of Oslo, and previous head of Gaustad Hospital, Oslo. His research includes studies in drug addiction, paranoid disorders, and personal follow-ups of suicide attempters. He was President of the International Association for Suicide Prevention (IASP) from 1988 to 1991. He is an honorary member of IASP and was awarded a prize by the organization in 1999 in recognition of his life's work.

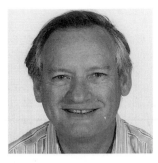

Alec Roy

Alec Roy, MD, is Professor of Psychiatry at the New Jersey Medical School. His main area of research is suicidology, especially risk factors, genetics, alcohol and substance dependence, schizophrenia, depression and prevention. He received the Louis Dublin Award of the American Association of Suicidology and the Stengel Research Award of the International Association for Suicide Prevention in 1999.

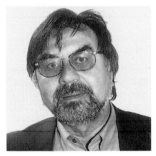

Wolfgang Rutz

Associate Professor Wolfgang Rutz holds an MD from the University of Würzburg and a PhD from the University of Linkøping, Sweden. He was director of mental health services on Gotland for many years and has been intensively engaged in the development of mental health services in Sweden and the Nordic and Baltic countries. Over the last decade his research has focussed on the prevention and monitoring of depressive conditions and suicidality. In 1998 Dr Rutz was appointed Regional Adviser for Mental Health at the WHO Regional Office for Europe in Copenhagen.

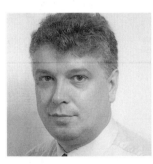

Paul Salkovskis

Paul Salkovskis is Professor of Cognitive Psychology at Oxford University and Honorary Consultant Clinical Psychologist for Oxford District Mental Health Trust, Oxford, UK. In 1990 Professor Salkovskis collaborated in a controlled trial using cognitive behavioural therapy in repeated suicide cases at Leeds General Infirmary. He took up a new post at the Institute of Psychiatry, London, in October 2000.

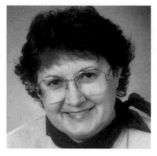

Sylvia Schaller

Sylvia Schaller, PhD, is a clinical psychologist and psychotherapist. She is Deputy Head of the Outpatient Clinic of the Otte-Selz-Institute, University of Mannheim, Germany, where she is also Lecturer at the Faculty of Social Sciences and Lecturer and Supervisor in behaviour therapy. Her research interests include behavioural therapy, suicide and attitudes towards assisted suicide in the elderly, and personality disorders.

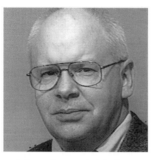

Armin Schmidtke

Armin Schmidtke, PhD, is Professor and a clinical psychologist and psychotherapist. He is a lecturer at the Faculty of Philosophy and Head of the Department of Clinical Psychology at the Clinic for Psychiatry and Psychotherapy, University of Würzburg, Germany. Professor Schmidtke is President of the International Academy for Suicide Research, and temporary adviser for suicidology of the World Health Organization. He is the recipient of the first Hans-Rost award from the German Association for Suicide Prevention (1998), and the 1997 winner of the Stengel Research Award from the international Association for Suicide Prevention. Professor Schmidtke's research interests include behavioural therapy, single case statistics, suicidology, and the effect of the media.

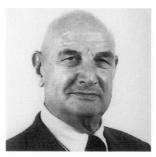

Jean-Pierre Soubrier

Jean-Pierre Soubrier, MD, is Professor at the Collège de Médecine des Hôpitaux de Paris, France, Chief Psychiatrist at University Hospital Cochin (Paris, AP-HP). His research career began in 1965 as a Fulbright Research Fellow at the Suicide Prevention Center, Los Angeles, USA. He is the Founding President of the Groupement d'Etudes et de Prévention du Suicide, France, and Past President of the International Association for Suicide Prevention (IASP). He is WHO Advisor to the Global Network for Suicide Prevention and Research. His awards include the Silver Medal from the Faculty of Medicine, Paris (1965); the Stengel Award, IASP (1981); and the Annual Award from Académie Nationale de Médecine, France (1985). Professor Soubrier is European Editor of the journal *Suicide and Life-threatening Behaviour* (USA).

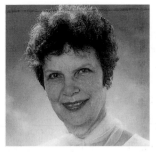

Airi Värnik

Airi Värnik, MD, PhD, Professor of Social Psychiatry at Tartu University, graduated as a psychiatrist from Tartu University, Estonia. Her first doctoral thesis from the Leningrad Behterev Institute examined presenile psychoses, while her second thesis from the Karolinska Institute was on the epidemiology of suicide in the former USSR. Dr Värnik is a founder and Director of the Estonian-Swedish Institute of Suicidology in Tallinn.

Foreword

Suicide is a public health problem. A cold look at figures indicates that approximately one million people take their own lives every year around the world. But this does not reveal all; it does not tell us about the suffering of relatives, friends and colleagues left behind, often puzzled and disturbed by that extreme act of self-destruction, often stigmatized.

Of great concern is a recent increase of suicide rates among young people; nowadays the largest proportion of committed suicides relates to people below the age of 45 years. Another major concern is linked to other forms of suicidal behaviour, e.g., suicide attempts, which represent a major burden on the health-care system, particularly on emergency rooms.

And yet, a large proportion of suicidal behaviour can be prevented, particularly those cases associated with mental disorders, a majority, in fact. We have now hard evidence about efficient methods for preventing suicide; it is regrettable that only a handful of health authorities have realized the economic and human burden created by suicide and have accordingly adopted policies and lunched programmes for the prevention of suicide.

WHO, as the major international organization in the field of health, has recognized the public health importance of suicide by adopting recently a strategy for raising awareness of authorities, decision makers, professionals and the public at large about this problem. It is also prepared, through its own resources and its network of Collaborating Centres and individual experts to provide technical assistance to countries willing to develop programmes and activities for the prevention of suicide.

In view of the large proportion of people with mental disorder who make attempts against their own lives WHO's Department of Mental Health and Substance Dependence has taken the lead for the co-ordination activities related to the prevention of suicide. We are happy to see this book come to light. Some of its contributors are members of the WHO network of experts on suicidology and we are confident that with their help we can effectively make a difference in this domain.

Dr Benedetto Saraceno
Director
Department of Mental Health and Substance Dependence
World Health Organization
Geneva
Switzerland

Foreword

When I first started my research in suicide prevention over 50 years ago the taboo surrounding suicide was recognized early as a major hurdle blocking our efforts at suicide prevention – impeding identification, assessment and treatment. It was also clear that overcoming this hurdle could be accomplished only by much targeted education and information. It is astounding how much in a mere half century the field of suicide has sprung to life and burgeoned, with what is now a vast number of related publications, research and clinical centers, plays and films. All of these have helped to overcome the general unwillingness to openly discuss and examine the subject.

Though difficult to measure or to quantify, there is no doubt in my mind that the taboo surrounding suicide has diminished. Nevertheless, cultural and religious precepts in many countries continue to play an important role in attitudes toward suicide, and often still keep it from being mentioned even when it occurs within the family. Of course, we do not want to erase all the taboos around suicide – which often act as a deterrent in a moment of overwhelming stress – rather alter perceptions just enough to allow suicidal people to ask for help, now so much more available than when we first started. This at least allows significant others to hear, to listen, and to prevent what Professor Wasserman has so aptly used to title this welcome publication – an unnecessary death.

Suicide: an unnecessary death is a delight to read – it is as simple and direct as possible, yet includes all the major areas of current concern and interest in the field. Professor Wasserman has written for an important audience that until now has been virtually ignored. This book is not directed at the professional suicidologist/researcher/clinician (although they would also profit greatly from reading it); rather it is directed at the 'busy clinician' who is dealing with the patient in many different every day circumstances. *Suicide: an unnecessary death* will also be welcomed by groups such as the police, probation officers and teachers who will benefit from a facilitated introduction to the entire field of suicide prevention.

I predict that this book will be of much use and interest to others, as it already has been to me.

Professor Norman L Farberow
Los Angeles, CA
USA

Preface

Approximately one million people worldwide commit suicide every year, and at least ten times as many attempt suicide. A considerable number of these are in contact with the health-care sector. Encounters with suicidal individuals are therefore common in the everyday work of health-care staff.

A massive expansion is under way in psychiatric research. This applies to every field, including suicidology. There has therefore been a constant increase in the number of articles and books reporting research findings about suicide and attempted suicide.

The abundance of new literature makes it difficult for busy clinicians, GPs, counsellors, volunteers and other staff whose clinical practice involves daily contact with suicidal patients to devote sufficient time to penetrating this literature and, accordingly, apply new findings in their clinical practice. Moreover, health-care services in almost every country have undergone restructuring and various cost-cutting measures that, in turn, have reduced the time available to health-care staff for their own education. This is the background to this book as a summary of the latest findings that may be useful to practitioners.

The aim of this book is to convey to the reader the vast experience of research and clinical work gained by leading experts in the field of suicidology who joined me in this effort. For didactic reasons, all chapters are written in discursive, textbook style, rather than in the style of a scientific paper. Consequently, the number of references carefully selected by the authors is limited. Early findings are usually reported in the references listed in the book. Each chapter is also of limited length to provide a rapid overview for health-care staff, who work under heavy time and emotional pressure, of the assessment and treatment methods recommended for daily use.

The book is directed at clinical psychiatrists and other physicians, as well as other staff who work with psychiatric patients, but who have no implicit knowledge of the field of suicidology.

In the prevention of suicidal acts, the patient's compliance with both pharmaceutical and psychotherapeutic treatment is paramount. In this context, the psychodynamics between the suicidal patient and their family, significant others and care providers are crucial. Treatment of the suicidal patient can succeed only if the health-care staff concerned are aware of their own attitudes and their impact on the suicidal patients and their family, and also of the psychosocial stressors that cannot be treated with psychiatric methods.

Psychiatric treatment involving a combination of pharmacological and psychotherapeutic methods must always be supplemented by various psychosocial measures. Professionals outside the health-care sector, as well as the families, friends and colleagues and workmates where available, should be involved in implementing these measures. If we professionals in the health care sector remain aware of these aspects, it will make our clinical practice more effective and easier.

This book represents the latest developments in suicidology research, and draws on the experience of a wide range of international experts. Should any reader have comments on the issues discussed, their views would be welcomed at suicid.forskning@ipm.ki.se

I wish to acknowledge the enthusiastic and considerable support I have received, in the course of preparing this book, from all the contributors and their administrative staff. I would also like to thank my husband Professor Jerzy Wasserman, who read all the manuscripts, and was an unfailing and inspiring discussion partner throughout.

Professor Danuta Wasserman
Director
Swedish National Centre for Suicide Research
and Prevention of Mental Ill-Health
Stockholm
Sweden

Section I
Epidemiology

Suicide in the world: latest available date. Source: WHO Mortality Database.

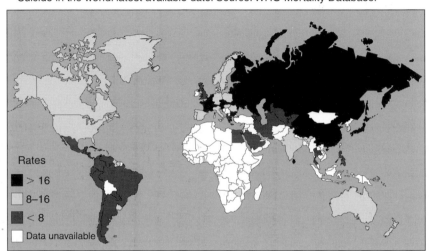

■ High suicide rates. From 16−46 per cent per 100,000 of the population and over.

▢ Intermediate suicide rates. From 8−16 per 100,000 of the population.

■ Low suicide rates. Under 8 per 100,000 of the population.

▢ Data not available.

1
Suicide in the world: an epidemiological overview 1959–2000

José M Bertolote

Information sources

One of the constitutional functions of the World Health Organization (WHO) is the collation and dissemination of data on mortality and morbidity. Since its creation in 1948, WHO has been collaborating with its member states with a view to perfecting methods for obtaining, processing and analysing these data. As a result, WHO maintains a data bank on mortality in which deaths from all causes are reported by member states, usually split by sex and age. The information is reported to WHO as the actual number of deaths in each demographic category and is then transformed into rates. The WHO data bank on mortality has grown from 33 member states in the early 1950s to some 130 member states currently.

Of special relevance to the field of suicidology, most countries include information on mortality associated with suicide, the category name and code of which has remained relatively stable through successive editions of the International Classification of Causes of Death (ICD), from ICD-6 in 1950 to ICD-10. The most recent data available are shown in Table 1.1.[1]

Whenever figures on suicide are presented or discussed there is always the question of their reliability, since in some instances – and for several reasons – suicide as a reason for death can be hidden; therefore, real figures may be higher. This point is acknowledged, which only reinforces the gravity of the global picture of suicide. Another question that is frequently raised refers to the comparability of data across countries. The information presented here reflects the official figures made available to WHO by its member states; these, in turn, are based on real death certificates signed by legally authorized personnel, usually doctors and, to a lesser extent, police officers. Generally speaking, these professionals do not misrepresent the information, and the real dimension of eventual distortions introduced by misreporting remains to be demonstrated. It is my hope that these figures can provide a solid ground against which corrections and improvements can be brought about.

Table 1.1   Suicide rates by country (per 100,000 population) (most recent year available).

Country	Year	Men	Women
Albania	1993	2.9	1.7
Argentina	1993	10.6	2.9
Armenia	1992	3.6	1.0
Australia	1995	19.0	5.1
Austria	1997	30.0	10.0
Azerbaijan	1996	1.5	0.3
Bahamas	1995	2.2	0.0
Bahrain	1988	4.9	0.5
Barbados	1995	9.5	3.7
Belarus	1993	48.7	9.6
Belgium	1992	26.7	11.0
Belize	1995	12.0	0.9
Brazil	1992	5.6	1.6
Bulgaria	1994	25.3	9.7
Canada	1995	21.5	5.4
Chile	1994	10.2	1.4
China (Hong Kong)	1995	14.3	9.2
China (mainland)	1994	14.3	17.9
Colombia	1994	5.5	1.5
Costa Rica	1994	8.0	1.8
Croatia	1996	34.2	11.3
Cuba	1995	25.6	14.9
Czech Republic	1996	24.0	6.8
Denmark	1996	24.3	9.8
Dominican Republic	1994	0.0	0.0
Ecuador	1995	6.4	3.2
Egypt	1987	0.1	0.0
El Salvador	1990	15.6	7.7
Estonia	1996	64.3	14.1
Finland	1995	43.4	11.8
France	1995	30.4	10.8
Georgia	1990	5.4	2.0
Germany	1997	22.1	8.1
Greece	1996	5.7	1.2
Guatemala	1984	0.9	0.1
Guyana	1994	14.6	6.5
Honduras	1976	0.0	0.0
Hungary	1997	49.2	15.6
Iceland	1995	16.4	3.8
India	1995	11.4	8.0
Iran	1991	0.3	0.1
Ireland	1995	17.9	4.6
Israel	1996	8.2	2.6
Italy	1993	12.7	4.0
Jamaica	1985	0.5	0.2
Japan	1996	24.3	11.5
Jordan	1979	0.0	0.0
Kazakhstan	1996	51.9	9.5

Kuwait	1994	1.8	1.9
Kyrgyzstan	1996	17.6	3.8
Latvia	1996	64.3	13.5
Lithuania	1996	79.3	17.1
Luxembourg	1997	29.0	9.8
Malta	1997	5.9	2.1
Mauritius	1996	20.6	6.4
Mexico	1995	5.4	1.0
Netherlands	1995	13.1	6.5
New Zealand	1994	23.6	5.8
Nicaragua	1994	4.7	2.2
Norway	1995	19.1	6.2
Panama	1987	5.6	1.9
Paraguay	1994	3.4	1.2
Peru	1989	0.6	0.4
Philippines	1993	2.5	1.7
Poland	1996	24.1	4.6
Portugal	1996	10.3	3.1
Puerto Rico	1992	16.1	1.9
Qatar	1995	0.0	0.0
Republic of Korea	1995	14.5	6.7
Republic of Moldova	1996	30.9	6.2
Romania	1996	21.3	4.3
Russian Federation	1995	72.9	4.3
Saint Kitts and Nevis	1995	0.0	0.0
Saint Lucia	1986–1988	11.0	3.0
Saint Vincent and Grenadines	1982–1985	2.0	0.0
Sao Tome and Principe	1984–1985	3.7	0.0
Seychelles	1985–1987	12.2	0.0
Singapore	1997	14.3	8.0
Slovakia	1995	23.4	4.6
Slovenia	1996	48.0	13.9
Spain	1995	12.5	3.7
Sri Lanka	1995	44.6	16.8
Suriname	1992	16.6	7.2
Sweden	1996	20.0	8.5
Switzerland	1994	30.9	12.2
Syrian Arab Republic	1985	0.2	0.0
Tajikistan	1992	5.1	2.3
Thailand	1994	5.6	2.4
Trinidad and Tobago	1994	17.4	5.0
Turkmenistan	1994	8.1	3.4
UK	1997	11.0	3.2
Ukraine	1992	38.2	9.2
Uruguay	1990	16.6	4.2
USA	1996	19.3	4.4
Uzbekistan	1993	9.3	3.2
Venezuela	1994	8.3	1.9
Zimbabwe	1990	10.6	5.2

Source: World Health Organization.

Suicide rates

According to WHO estimates for the year 2020, approximately 1.53 million people will die from suicide, and 10–20 times more people than this will attempt suicide worldwide. This represents on average one death every 20 seconds and one attempt every 1–2 seconds.

Although it is customary in the suicidology literature to present rates of suicide for both men and women combined (the so called total suicide rates), it should be noted that the current general epidemiological practice is to present rates according to sex and age, particularly when important differences (in terms of figures or of risk factors) across sex or age groups exist. This is precisely the situation in relation to suicide (suicide rates of men and women are consistently different in most places, as are rates in different age groups). Therefore, data are presented in Table 1.1 by sex; this information is later disaggregated by age for some analytical considerations.

A close inspection of Table 1.1 reveals that the highest suicide rates for both men and women are found in Europe, more particularly in Eastern Europe, in a group of countries that share similar genetic, historical and sociocultural characteristics, such as Estonia, Latvia, Lithuania and, to a lesser extent, Finland, Hungary and the Russian Federation. Nevertheless, some similarly high rates are also found in countries that are quite distinct in relation to these characteristics, such as Sri Lanka and Cuba.

Curiously enough, when the data are separated by WHO region, the highest rates in each region with the exception of Europe, are found in island countries, such as Cuba, Japan, Mauritius and Sri Lanka. Also, according to the WHO regional distribution, the lowest rates as a whole are found in the eastern Mediterranean Region, which comprises mostly countries that follow Islamic traditions; this is also true of some Central Asian republics that were formerly integrated in the Soviet Union.

From Table 1.1 it can also be seen that with only one exception (China) suicide rates in males are consistently higher than suicide rates in females.

In Figure 1.1, global suicide rates (per 100,000 population) have been calculated starting from 1950: deaths reported by countries in each year were averaged and projected in relation to the global population over 5 years of age at each respective year. An increase of approximately 49% for suicide rates in males and 33% for suicide rates in females can be observed between 1950 and 1995; this graph also highlights the relatively constant predominance of suicide rates in males over suicide rates in females: 3.2:1 in 1950, 3.6:1 in 1995 and 3.9:1 in 2020.

The increase in these global suicide rates must be interpreted with caution. On the one hand, it might reflect the fact that since the end of the USSR (which had an overall rate below the average), some of its former republics (particularly those with the highest rates in the world) started to report indi-

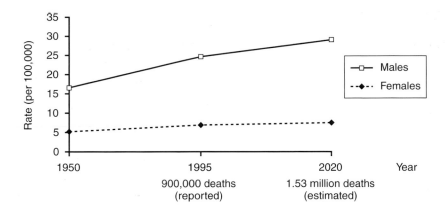

Figure 1.1

Global suicide rates since 1950 and trends until 2020.

vidually, thus inflating the global rate. On the other hand, figures for 1950 were based on 21 countries only, and this gradually increased up to 1995, when the estimates are based on 105 countries that now report on causes of death. These 105 countries as a whole probably have higher rates, are more concerned with them and have a higher tendency to report on suicide mortality than countries where suicide is not perceived as a major public health problem.

As for age, there is a clear tendency for suicide rates to increase with age (Figure 1.2). Against an average global suicide rate of 24.7 deaths per 100,000 for men, the rates for specific age groups start at 0.9 (in the age

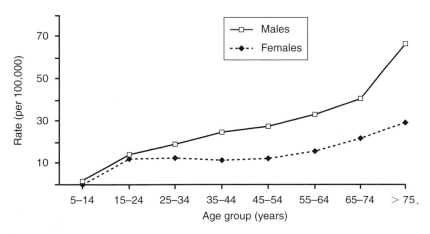

Figure 1.2

Global suicide rates by sex and age in selected countries.

group 5–14 years) and gradually increase up to 66.9 (in the age group over 75 years). The same positive relationship between age and suicide rates is observed in relation to suicide rates in females: for an overall rate of 6.9, specific age group rate grow from 0.5 per 100,000 (in the age group 5–14 years) to 29.7 (in the age group over 75 years).

Suicide frequency

In spite of the wide (and appropriate use) of rates, the information conveyed by them alone can be misleading, particularly when comparing data across countries or regions with important differences in demographic structure. As indicated earlier, the highest suicide rates are currently found in Eastern Europe; however, the largest number of suicides takes place in Asia. Table 1.2 compares the ranking of the top 10 countries in terms of both the frequency of suicides and the calculated suicide rates.

Of the total number of successful suicides worldwide, approximately 45% take place in those ten countries in the left hand column of Table 1.2. Conversely, the top 10 countries in terms of rates (right hand part of Table 1.2) represent less than 8% of all completed suicides. Two countries, namely China and India, are responsible for almost 30% of all cases of suicide committed worldwide, although the suicide rate of China practically coincides with the global average and that of India is almost half of the global suicide rate. The number of suicides in China alone is 30% greater than the total number of suicides in the whole of Europe, and the number of suicides in India alone (the second highest) is equivalent to those in the four European countries with the highest number of suicides together (Russia, Germany, France and Ukraine).

Only two countries – the Russian Federation and Sri Lanka – are among the top 10 countries by both suicide rate and number of cases of suicide. The other eight countries in the top 10 by number of suicides all rank below the 11th position by rate; one (Brazil, ninth by number of suicides) ranks 71st by rate. Conversely, the other eight countries in the top 10 by rate rank below the 14th position by number of suicides.

Given the relatively narrow differences in the population of males and females in each age group, the large predominance of suicide rates among males is also found in relation to the actual number of suicides committed.

It is in relation to age, however, that the most striking changes in the picture are perceived when we move from rates to frequency. Although suicide rates can be between six and eight times higher among the elderly compared with young people, currently more young people than elderly people are dying from suicide, globally speaking (Table 1.3). Currently, more suicides (53%) are committed by people aged 5–44 years than by people aged 45 years and more (Figure 1.3). Also, the age group in which most suicides are currently completed is 35–44 years for both men and women.

Table 1.2   Ranking of the top 10 countries for total number of suicides (estimated for the year 2000) and total suicide rates (most recent year available).

Country	Number of suicides	Rate per 100,000	Ranking by number of suicides	Country	Number of suicides	Rate per 100,000	Ranking by suicide rate
China	195,000	16.1	24	Lithuania	1,600	45.6	22
India	87,000	9.7	45	Russia	57,800	41.5	3
Russia	57,800	41.5	2	Latvia	1,000	40.7	23
USA	31,000	11.9	38	Estonia	600	40.1	25
Japan	20,000	16.8	23	Finland	1,700	33.8	21
Germany	12,500	22.6	11	Hungary	3,000	32.9	16
France	11,600	15.8	25	Sri Lanka	5,400	31.0	9
Ukraine	11,000	20.7	14	Kazakhstan	4,500	28.6	13
Brazil	5,400	3.5	71	Belarus	2,800	28.0	17
Sri Lanka	5,400	31.0	7	Slovenia	600	26.6	24

Source: World Health Organization.

Table 1.3   Percentage of suicides by age group and sex in selected countries* (most recent year available).

Age (years)	5–14	15–24	25–34	35–44	45–54	55–64	65–74	.75	Total
Men	0.7	12.7	18.3	20.5	17	13.9	9.6	7.3	100
Women	0.9	13.3	15	15.4	14.7	13.9	13.7	13.1	100

Source: World Health Organization.
*Countries as in Table 1.2; does not include India.

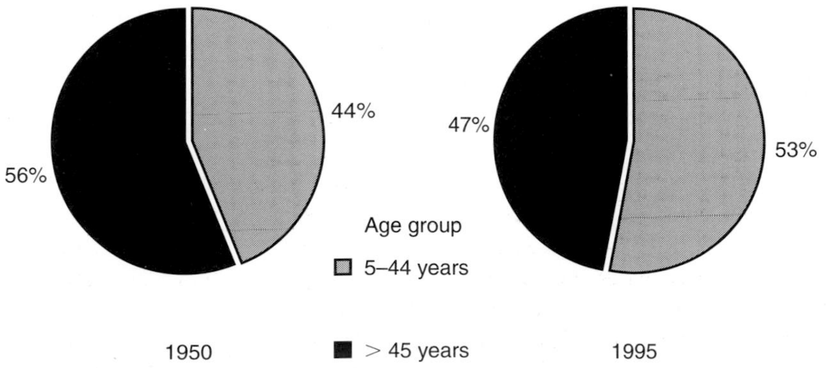

44%   47%
53%
56%

Age group
5–44 years

1950   > 45 years   1995

Figure 1.3
Suicides by age in selected countries (1950 and 1995).

This 'ungreying' of suicide is a relatively new phenomenon (Figure 1.3). It acquires a dramatic aspect when one considers that the proportion of the elderly in the total population is increasing at a greater rate than that of younger people. Also, it is not the result of a divergent modification in suicide rates in these age groups: the suicide rate in young people is increasing at a greater pace than it is in the elderly.

Methods of suicide

Although a good knowledge of the methods used for committing suicide is fundamental for suicide prevention programmes,[2] this is particularly relevant at the local level. On a global basis it is mostly of academic interest. Therefore, global data about methods used committing suicide are not presented here. Nevertheless, people involved with suicide prevention programmes are strongly urged to obtain as precise information about method and means of suicide as possible in order to improve the efficiency of those programmes (see Chapter 30).

Prevention of suicide

Global figures and statistics are very suitable for giving a broad view of a problem, raising awareness about it and providing a means of comparison with other problems. However, they hide important regional and local characteristics. Therefore, nothing can replace a sound local system for monitoring suicide trends, including methods of suicide and sociodemographic, psychiatric and psychological variables.

It is, nevertheless, hoped that the information provided here can both inform those interested in the subject and raise the interest and awareness of those who have not yet acknowledged the huge public health and personal burden represented by suicide.

References

1. World Health Organization. Figures and Facts about Suicide (Doc. WHO/MNH/MBD/99.1). WHO: Geneva, 1999.

2. World Health Organization. Primary prevention of mental, neurological and psychosocial disorders. WHO: Geneva, 1998.

Section II
Theoretical model of suicide behaviour

2
A stress–vulnerability model and the development of the suicidal process

Danuta Wasserman

Stress–vulnerability model

The causes of suicide are complex and no simple explanations of the phenomenon exist. Many people suffer from mental illnesses of various types, have personality disorders and have undergone terrible life events but nonetheless have neither considered taking their own lives nor committed such an act. The propensity to suicide has fascinated many researchers, and various models have been devised to explain the origins of suicidal behaviour.

In a comprehensive stress–diathesis model presented by Mann et al.,[1] genetic make-up as well as acquired susceptibility contributes to a person's constitutional predisposition or diathesis. Early traumatic life experiences, chronic illness (especially of the central nervous system), chronic alcohol and substance abuse, and also factors such as possibly cholesterol all play a part in the development of this diathesis. A diathesis for suicidal behaviour is held to be the crucial determinant of whether suicidality is manifested under the influence of stress as a result of, for example, acute psychiatric or somatic illness, severe abuse of alcohol and drugs, pressing social problems or family crises. Whether people take their own lives in such situations is thus explained with reference to variations in diathesis.

Neuropsychobiology and suicidal behaviour

The neurotransmitters of the brain are involved in regulating human physical and psychological functioning.[2-4] Experimental studies of animals and observation of people who have incurred brain damage, been subjected to neurosurgery or taken medication that affects various neurotransmitter systems have revealed that anxiety, aggression, pain perception and appetite are regulated by serotonin, while noradrenaline (norepinephrine) is involved in such functions as arousal, attention, processing of information and memory. The dopamine system, on the other hand, regulates cognition, reward and sexual behaviour.

Mood, emotions and cognitive functions are influenced by all three monoamine systems which interact in a complex manner, which means that a single function may be regulated by more than one neurotransmitter. If the action of a single neurotransmitter is stimulated, it is enough to attain effects in other systems as well.

Serotonin

The serotonergic system, which is substantially under genetic control and the activity of which shows considerable stability over time, is less state-dependent and more of a marker for a trait. It has been shown to be related to vulnerability to, or a diathesis for, suicidal behaviour (see Chapter 3). The effects of upbringing are superimposed on the genetic make-up and also on the serotonin system. Severe traumas due to deprivation during childhood may possibly reset serotonergic function, and this effect persists and may contribute to elevated suicide risk in later life.[5] Brain functions that were unaffected before a trauma may be modified as a result of the trauma.

Noradrenaline

Research findings about noradrenaline are less consistent than those relating to serotonin in terms of diathesis for suicidal behaviour. The noradrenaline system reacts more to acute stress and tends to state-dependent rather than trait-dependent (unlike the serotonin system). The noradrenaline system, too, is subject to genetic control and affected by environmental factors. Several observations indicate overactivity of the noradrenaline system and hyperactive stress response in suicidal patients.

Dopamine

Too few studies of dopamine in suicidal patients have been carried out, and its role in suicidal behaviour remains to be ascertained.

Stress

The connections between biological, psychosocial, cultural and environmental factors are a new and exciting field for research in suicidology. The balance between different neurotransmitters is a prerequisite for normal brain function and, accordingly, for our mental health.[6] Both acute and chronic stress caused by recurrent pressures in life result in changes in the concentrations of noradrenaline and Its receptors. The noradrenaline system, in turn, affects both the dopamine and the serotonin system, and so imbalance between the various neurotransmitters may arise.

Examples of current life situations and events that induce stress are severe crises, traumas, acute somatic or psychiatric illness, abuse, bereavement and separation from loved ones, unemployment, bullying or victimization, harassment at school or the workplace, and narcissistic injuries of various types (see Chapter 13). The person who experiences stress is then overwhelmed by anxiety, anger, sorrow, despondency and hopelessness, associated with marked physiological reactions. Repeated and lasting trauma makes people more susceptible, impairing their ability to cope with subsequent negative life events.[7,8]

Lack of sleep, seasonal darkness, misuse of alcohol and drugs as well as inadequate diet contribute to a person's susceptibility (diathesis), since these circumstances affect neurotransmitter synthesis and function.

Interactions between different neurotransmitters, stress hormones and other hormones, and the immune system is receiving increasing attention, as are the influences of painful experiences in early life and adulthood.[9] Early traumas affect how the 'psychoneurohormonal' systems of the brain react to mental and social stress in later life. In a person who has been subjected to long-term stress and trauma, renewed stress may disturb a range of biological reactions. People suffering from stress not only show manifestations of various mental illnesses more readily but also succumb to infections, muscular pain and similar ailments more easily than other people. Even recollections of earlier stressful situations – torture, separations and other traumas – can provoke reactions that involve both physical and mental symptoms.

Reactions to stress which involve the hypothalamic–pituitary–adrenal (HPA) axis are dependent on both inherited and acquired factors and may be more or less labile. Animal experiments have shown that in juvenile rats that undergo early separation from their mothers, which implies a considerable stress, the cortisol system is unstable.[10] That the same applies to human beings is highly probable. The results of several surveys relating to the HPA axis show that the presence of chronic distress may contribute to suicide risk.[11,12] An increase of corticotrophin-releasing hormone produced in the hypothalamus and corticosteroids disregulate both noradrenaline and serotonin activity.

Stress may make suicidal people forget adequate coping strategies

The connections between stress, stress hormones and memory have now been demonstrated experimentally.[13] The healthy subjects treated with cortisone, which is rapidly converted into cortisol in the body, were found to have difficulty in memorizing verbal material. It is well known that stress in conjunction with examinations may make students forget their knowledge. Once the examination is over and they have calmed down, they suddenly remember how they should have answered.

The same may be true of suicidal people. In situations of stress, their capacity to act and their cognition are severely impaired. If these have been poor from the start owing to innate vulnerability and the additional susceptibility acquired during childhood, there may not be much room for manoeuvre when another stressful situation is encountered in later life.[14]

Does the noradrenaline system fail in suicide patients?

Studies of polymorphism in a specific gene that codes for (i.e. governs the production of) an enzyme known as tyrosin hydroxylase (TH), which participates in the synthesis of noradrenaline and dopamine, have been carried out by my research group.[15] The subjects were Swedish patients who had attempted suicide and mentally healthy controls. A particular variant (polymorphism) of the TH gene (a significant higher incidence of the allele TH-K3, also named T8) proved to be over-represented among certain patients who had attempted suicide, and also among non-suicidal subjects of a certain personality type. These results are preliminary and need further replication.

People with this allele were characterized by low stress tolerance and a tendency towards irritability, angry and hostility reactions as well as by vulnerability, measured by the NEO Personality Inventory, Revised version (NEO PI-R).[15] Interpreting these results is far from straightforward. One possibility may be that this variant of the gene results in smaller quantities of noradrenaline being released or in a lower turnover in the brains of suicidal people in comparison with others. Furthermore, noradrenaline is required to enable people to analyse incoming information and to function appropriately.

Suicidal subjects perceive that they have reached a point of no return and lose the ability to contemplate their lives in a balanced way. Rigid strategies are applied. This may be because the noradrenaline metabolism and the ability to refill brain depots of noradrenaline sufficiently fast at times of stress are, to some degree, defective in these people. This hypothesis may supplement the serotonin hypothesis described in Chapter 3. In situations of stress, a noradrenaline deficiency may therefore conceivably result in less well-considered reactions. When exposed to extreme stress due to, for example, negative life events, people with this disposition may be unable to find constructive ways out of the situation since their biological vulnerability (possibly owing to the above-mentioned polymorphism or other, yet unknown genetic defects) restricts the scope for recovery and the choice of alternative, more constructive strategies (see Chapter 14).

Offsetting the diathesis at an early stage

In suicide prevention, it is essential to detect individual vulnerability at an early stage in order to try to prevent exacerbation of this vulnerability during childhood and in adult life. This should preferably be done even at the stage of planning for pregnancy in a family with suicidal behaviour in the anamnesis, since the genetic component of suicide is well known. The purpose is to strengthen the parents' skills to enable them to make good health choices for themselves and for the child and to develop and adopt objectives in life that can be realized. It is hoped that the influence of genetic inheritance can be reduced by establishing optimal external circumstances.

Genetic inheritance is important but does not imply 'predestination'

Many people believe that genetic inheritance is important enough to preclude freedom of action, but this is far from true. All monozygotic twins have the same genetic make-up, but if one twin succumbs to depression there is approximately a 50–60% risk of the other also doing so. If one monozygotic twin dies from suicide, the risk of the other dying from suicide is only 13%.[16]

Biological vulnerability (an innate trait, part of the genetic make-up) is, in some people, exacerbated if the person grows up and lives in an unfavourable psychosocial environment.[17] It may then develop into a mental illness, which is an obvious risk factor for suicide. The same may occur during adulthood. When the environment is perceived as excessively stressful and the vulnerable person cannot cope with the external stress, the pressure becomes too heavy, and anxiety, depression, a sense of hopelessness and severe suicidal ideation, culminating in suicide, may ensue.

Change in brain structures

Various protective factors may conceivably affect brain function in a positive direction. Several studies show that the structures of the brain are well developed at birth, but also that they can be influenced in later life. Traumatic experiences, such as violence, incest and other highly unfavourable situations day after day for long periods in childhood impose severe stress. This stress affects structures in the brain, such as the hypothalamus and hypophysis, and also the adrenal glands, whose increased secretion of hormones (cortisol and adrenaline (epinephrine)) has an adverse impact on the central nervous system.[4] This may, in some cases, result in neuronal destruction in the hippocampus, which is the oldest part of the brain in evolutionary terms. It has long been known that the brain can be damaged, but neuroscience has recently yielded revolutionary findings that it also has a regeneration and repair capacity.[18,19]

Neurones can be re-formed and regenerated by means of increased cell division and cell growth, and new connections between brain cells can also develop. It is probable that favourable living circumstances can also leave their mark on the brain. Increased blood flow in the brain in conjunction with various forms of activity, including psychotherapy, has been described. The question has arisen of whether brain activity merely undergoes temporary modification or whether the change is more long-lasting. Can the patient conceivably acquire new neural connections or neurones? This seems to be the case and may eventually imply that psychosocial measures make people less vulnerable to stress, and give them greater influence over their own well-being.

The central nervous system is thus not as immutable as was previously believed. It is constantly developing, with close interactions between what we have inherited and what we acquire through interplay with our immediate surroundings, both psychosocial and physical. Nobody is therefore predestined to suicide.

Classification of suicidal behaviour

Suicide is, by definition, a deliberate act. But unconscious psychological components play an important part. If there is no farewell letter, it is sometimes difficult to know the reasons for a suicide and whether it was a deliberate step or accidental or the result of taking prescription drugs, alcohol or an overdose of narcotics without the intention of dying. Behind many suicides there is probably no real intention to die.

If the person survives, it is recorded as a suicide attempt. People who attempt suicide are, nonetheless, different from those who actually take their own lives, and the practice of describing them as two separate but overlapping populations persists. From an epidemiological perspective these two populations differ, although they may not differ so much from the psychological point of view. There are many suicide attempters who resemble people who commit suicide.

The dividing line between serious thoughts of suicide and suicide attempts is sometimes difficult to draw. Nonetheless, it is surprising how far the results of randomized studies from various population groups and countries tally in terms of past-year prevalence of suicidal thoughts (9–13%) and also of lifetime (3–5%) and past-year (0.2–0.6%) prevalence of attempted suicide.[20]

Pokorny[21] introduced the concept of suicidal behaviour to cover suicidal thoughts (suicidal ideation), attempted suicide and suicide. At the same time, Paykel et al.[22] introduced such concepts as weariness of life and death wishes. These could be regarded as phenomena distinct from, and forerunners to, suicidal thoughts. With these notions, the foundation was laid for the model of the suicidal process.

Beskow[23] took these concepts to the fore and developed the model that is frequently used in retrospective studies of completed suicides.

The model shows that suicidal behaviour has a previous history and that the current process is a continuum of gradually increasing serious-ness in suicidal behaviour, from weariness of life to death wishes, suici-dal thoughts, suicide attempts and suicide.

Wasserman's studies[24] show that most suicidal acts are preceded by a process, of varying length, in which the dynamics is highly individual. The suicidal process usually stretches over months, but for some people it lasts more than a year and for patients with chronic depression, schizo-phrenics or substance abusers it can be lifelong. For young people with adjustment disorders, its duration may be only a few days or weeks. Propensity for suicide may be acute, chronic or latent. For long periods, thoughts of suicide may be entirely absent, only to return in response to new strains.

The suicidal process in the broad context of the stress-vulnerability model

The stress–diathesis model[1] can be supplemented with the broader model of development of the suicidal process in order to provide a better understanding of the dynamics in the interaction between suicidal people and the people around them, and to be able to study the 'suicidal com-munication' (the dynamics between the suicidal individual and his/her family and other key persons) as well as interplay between inherited and aquired conditions (Fig. 2.1). The factors that are taken into account in this model include:

- the role of the suicidal person's cognitive style and personality;
- the role of environmental factors;
- the way in which stress contributes to the diathesis becoming manifest;
- how other people's reactions and psychosocial and cultural support can contribute to the outcome; and
- in which circumstances a person's vulnerability is held back (protective factors) and in which circumstances it is expressed in suicide or attempted suicide (risk factors).

In this model, the boundaries between suicidal thoughts and suicide attempts are no longer distinct but fluid. The outcome is affected by risk and protective factors in interaction with the diathesis. Suicide is regarded not as an illness but as an act stemming from the interplay between cogni-tive, affective and communicative aspects.

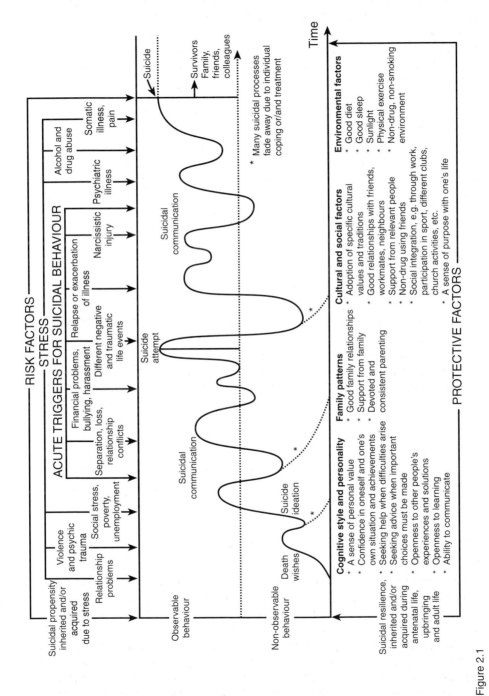

Figure 2.1

Stress-vulnerability model and development of the suicidal process from suicidal ideation to suicide. Wasserman D, 1999.

The suicidal process can be interrupted due to treatment but it may also abate spontaneously. The fact that the suicidal process is affected by numerous different factors is also suggested by various epidemiological surveys and individual psychological investigations. It is also vital to study the suicidal process not only at the individual level but also at the interpersonal (communicative) level and in relation to other external factors at the community level (in terms of social integration) as well as in relation to the cultural and the physical environment.

In this book, the term 'suicidal' is used to describe a person who has intense and serious thoughts about committing suicide. The term 'suicidal' also covers people who have less intensive or vague suicidal thoughts but are in the risk zone for suicide owing to various factors or who have attempted to take their own lives in the past year. These risk factors, include mental illness, personality disorder and negative life events (see Chapters 4 to 13). Risk is particularly high when one or more factors that normally afford a degree of protection (protective factors; discussed later in this chapter) are simultaneously eliminated.

Suicidal communication

The manner in which other people respond to a person's suicidal communication may afford some protection against suicidal behaviour.[24] Unfortunately, however, it may also be an obvious risk factor that adds to the chaos and self-hate experienced by the suicidal person, accelerating the suicidal process in a negative direction.[25] Whether the suicidal process is curtailed or proceeds to a suicide attempt or completed suicide depends on

- the person's capacity to ask for and receive help; and
- the capacity of other people (including staff) in the suicidal person's surroundings to recognize his or her suicidal communication and take it seriously.

Dialogue communication by suicidal people

Through dialogue and by using friendly words, one can help suicidal people to verbalize their elusive experiences and to convert them into words, which are the foundation of interpersonal communication and contact. To prevent suicidal people from resorting to suicide, it is important to take their every reference to suicide seriously.

The popular belief that people who talk about suicide do not commit it is a myth. However, there are some people on the verge of suicide who do not communicate their intentions. Although they may have partners, they are emotional loners and do not share their reflections with anyone.

After a suicide, the family may often express such thoughts as, 'I don't know who I was living with'. Men who live by the principle that strength lies in being alone and who neither wish nor dare to reveal their emotional needs and thoughts are well-known poor communicators. Young people, too, may have marked communication difficulties. People who communicate poorly may, on the surface, behave normally or almost normally while brooding intensely about suicide and planning the act.

Conversation as a means to reduce anxiety and chaos

Suicidal communication (i.e. references to thoughts about the act and plans to commit it) may vary sharply in intensity both over a day and in a longer perspective. By dialogue, a person may be diverted from thoughts of suicide and provided with some scope for alternative ways of solving conflicts. Other options suggested by the helper may perhaps be rejected at first but eventually absorbed and, possibly, applied. Conversation and communication reduce confusion, anxiety and panic. A sensitive interlocutor, one who does not exacerbate the suicidal patient's feelings of shame or guilt or give offence and who is prepared to provide practical assistance by, for example, telephoning the hospital or helping with something that has been neglected during the chaotic period, is needed. Such people can arrest the mental paralysis that suicidal people may experience in face of the slightest commitment. It is thus possible, by means of dialogue and practical support, to broaden a suicidal person's tunnel vision and loosen his or her cognitive constriction.

Types of suicidal communication

Suicidal communication may be classified as verbal and non-verbal. Both these types of communication can be further divided into direct and indirect communication.[24,25]

Direct verbal communication
In direct verbal suicidal communication, people directly express their intention to take their own lives or, less clearly, the feeling that everything is hopeless and the only right thing to do is to put an end to it all. This form of communication is sometimes expressed in quarrels, along with accusations directed at significant others – that they have caused difficulties, and, by implication, the suicidal situation.

Indirect verbal communication
Indirect verbal suicidal communication is sometimes less intelligible, since such utterances as, 'I can't go on like this', 'I don't see any point in living', 'Perhaps we won't see each other again' and 'It's hardly surprising

that lots of people want to kill themselves, the way society is' are often difficult to interpret. To be comprehensible, such messages need to be put in context. Some are easy to interpret; others can be understood only with hindsight.

Direct non-verbal communication
Examples of direct non-verbal suicidal communication may be the acquisition of a weapon or the collecting of drug prescriptions or medicines.

Indirect non-verbal communication
Writing a will, giving away keepsakes, paying debts and arranging insurance may be examples of indirect non-verbal suicidal communication. Intensive efforts to get in touch with loved ones or health-care services or to seek solitude and isolation may be other expressions of suicidal intent.

Response of significant others

Empathy of surrounding people
Direct suicidal communication is easier to interpret, but it is often mistrusted by the recipients, who doubt whether the person genuinely intends to take his or her own life. The indirect forms of suicidal communication are more difficult to understand for outsiders, but members of the immediate family often see how the person has changed and instinctively understand the communication. At best, those in proximity to the suicidal person can then become aware of the situation and, besides showing empathy, provide support and ensure that adequate care and professional help are obtained.

Ambivalence of surrounding people
Some people may react with concern, anxiety and silence. Ambivalence towards suicidal people, with the simultaneous wish to stay with them and to leave them, to seek help and to wait, may result. In extreme cases, people may show direct or indirect aggression towards the suicidal person in various ways. There can be a paradoxical interplay between the hypersensitive suicidal person, who is desperate, chaotic, irritable, sometimes aggressive, or paralysed in terms of coping strategies, and the surrounding people, who tend to be silent, cautious, withdrawn or show turning away reactions.

The reactions of which other people are capable have a crucial bearing on whether the development of the suicidal process is curtailed or accelerated. Their silence affords no help to a person who is suicidal. If they are ambivalent, the suicidal person's ambivalence may be reinforced and a vicious circle may arise. Suicidal individuals, owing to their disturbed perception, look on the dark side of everything, disparage themselves and magnify their own difficulties. They often perceive only the negative pole of family members' or other peoples' ambivalence (for example the expressions of the desire to break off the relationship or not to help) and they interpret these expressions as lack of love and interest and as rejection. They have difficulty in perceiving the positive pole of the ambivalence (for example the care and concern), although these sides are also very often present.

Aggression of surrounding people
If the relatives or significant others of a suicidal person become extremely frustrated and turn their backs or show aggression in verbal or non-verbal ways, the suicidal person is left to his or her own devices, alone with his or her own aggression, which can then be turned inwards. In some cases the suicidal person can be killed by the indifference or aggression of others which is directed towards them.

The life-saving actions of surrounding people

Other people's reactions have a particularly decisive impact when a suicidal person has only one relationship. The reactions of health-care personnel are equally important (see Chapters 17 and 27). Relatives and others who are close to those who are suicidal need (and deserve) a great deal of support and, sometimes, professional help, since their ambivalent and aggressive reactions stem from their own mental conflicts being brought to the fore when they find themselves in a situation of extreme duress.

Menninger, like Freud before him, saw suicide as a reflected murder, or 'inverted homicide'. Menninger believed that anger was turned inwards by the individual, instead of being expressed outwardly towards the individual responsible for the feeling of anger (see Chapter 14).

In-depth studies

The model presented in Figure 2.1 also provides scope for studying a suicidal person's fantasies, wishes and thoughts, intentions, plans, impulses and decisions to commit suicide. The stages of the suicidal process may be seen as attempts to resolve various internal psychic and external conflicts, to find new means of adjustment to an untenable life situation or to communicate a 'cry for help'.

The idea of suicide may at first be fleeting. It may be rejected, then return, only to be rejected once more . . . and so on until, eventually, it may appear to be the only option.

Immediately before the suicidal act (whether suicide attempt or suicide), the intensity of the suicidal process rises and feelings of hopelessness, helplessness and desperation are mixed with the symptoms of various psychiatric disorders. Similarly, the personality traits are accentuated. Inappropriate strategies for dealing with the life situation come to the fore when a person loses the capacity for taking an overall view, owing to drastically curtailed cognitive ability and 'blinkered vision'. Anxiety fuels the suicidal process and the mind revolves around thoughts of how and where death will come. All this is communicated frequently to others in various ways.

When a person takes the definite decision to die, all this chaos may be replaced by a phase of tranquillity that often misleads others. However, when protective factors are present, the outcome is often that the act is never committed.

Protective factors

Risk, but also the presence or absence of the protective factors, determines whether people lose control over their life situation and whether the outcome is a suicide, an attempted suicide or merely suicidal thoughts. Suicidal ideation is situation-dependent, and suicidal acts occur only when risk factors are present and acting in concert and protective factors have disappeared.

Consequently, what makes the difference between life and death, however, is not only the presence of risk factors, but also access to protective factors that strengthen the suicidal person's coping strategies.

Protective factors may be connected with sources of pleasure that are not currently available but may return or, similarly, rewarding contacts, employment or interesting occupations. Other examples are rediscovering ties with the family – parents, siblings, children or grandchildren – and neighbours, and rejoining a religious, political, or other group. Finding a responsive person who is prepared to listen, and therapy and medication that may help to make accessible the coping strategies that a person has used successfully in the past, are other ways of strengthening suicide-preventive factors.

Protective factors are contained both in the minds of suicidal people and in their surroundings. Nowadays, research focuses on finding the long-term lifestyles that protect people against any suicidal behaviour. Cognitive flexibility, collecting information about the problem, finding alternative solutions, minimizing rather than exaggerating the significance of one's negative life situation, hopefulness, and the propensity of the suicidal person and his or her family to seek help are protective factors. On the other hand, blame, guilt and avoidance of problems are correlated with suicide risk.[14]

A protective lifestyle is the product of growing up in a secure setting, with continuity in terms of adequate parent figures who are emotionally responsive to the child's needs, values and norms and who care for the child from birth to adulthood.[26] This security is supplemented in due course by firm friendships, other adult networks, marriage and a new family. A social, cultural or religious context with the experience of meaning for the family and the individual's life is another protective factor.

Protective factors are essential for building sufficiently strong defences against suicidal impulses. Such protective factors also include treatment of any mental disorder that is present. The physical environment also plays a part in mental well-being, and a balanced diet and adequate sleep and light (all of which affect neurotransmitter function, and thus mental health), along with other environmental psycho-social factors, are other key protective factors.

References

1. Mann JJ, Waternaux C, Haas G, Malone K. Toward a clinical model of suicidal behaviour in psychiatric patients. *Am J Psychiatry* 1999;**156:**181–189.

2. Damasio AR. Towards a neuropathology of emotion and mood. *Nature* 1997;**386:**769–770.

3. Deakin JF. The role of serotonin in panic, anxiety and depression (review). *Int Clin Psychopharmacol* 1998;Suppl **4:**S1–S5.

4. Salloway S, Malloy P, Cummings JL (eds). The neuropsychiatry of limbic and subtropical disorders. *American Psychiatric Press* 1997.

5. Wilson J, Prabucki K. Stress sensitivity and psychopathology. In Wilson J (ed). Trauma, transformation and healing: an integrative approach to theory: research, and post-traumatic therapy. New York: Brunner–Mazel; 1989:75–110.

6. Kolb B, Whishaw IQ. Fundamentals of human neuropsychology. New York, WH Freeman and Company, 1995.

7. Adams D, Lehnert K. Prolonged trauma and subsequent suicidal behaviour: child abuse and combat trauma reviewed. *J Traumatic Stress* 1997;**10:**619–634.

8. Amir M, Kaplan Z, Efroni R, Kotler M. Suicide risk and coping styles in posttraumatic stress disorder patients. *Psychother Psychosom* 1999;**68:**76–81.

9. van der Kolk BA, Perry C, Herman JL. Childhood origins of self-destructive behavior. *Am J Psychiatry* 1991;**148:**1665–1671.

10. Liu D, Diorio J, Tannenbaum B, et al. Maternal care, hippocampal glucocorticoid receptors, and hypothalamic-pituitary-adrenal responses to stress. *Science* 1997;**277:**1659–1662.

11. Coccaro EF, Astill JL. Central serotonergic function in parasuicide. *Prog Neuropsychopharmacol Biol Psychiatry* 1990;**14:**663–674.

12. van Praag HM. Comorbidity (psycho) analysed. *Br J Psychiatry Suppl* 1996;**30:**129–134.

13. Newcomer JW, Selke G, Melson AK, et al. Decreased memory performance in healthy humans induced by stress-level cortisol treatment. *Archives of General Psychiatry.* 1999; **56(6):**527–533.

14. Horesh N, Rolnick T, Iancu I, et al. Coping styles and suicide risk. *Acta Psychiatr Scand* 1996;**93:**489–493.

15. Persson ML, Wasserman D, Geijer T, et al. Tyrosine hydroxylase allelic distribution in suicide attempters. *Psychiatry Res* 1997;**72:**73–80.

16. Roy A. Genetic and biologic risk factors for suicide in depressive disorders. *Psychiatric Quarterly* 1993;64:345–358.

17. Rubenstein JL, Halton A, Kasten

L, et al. Suicidal behaviour in adolescents: stress and protection in different family contexts. *Am J Orthopsychiatry* 1998;**68:**274–284.

18. Gage FH. Mammalian neural stem cells. *Science* 2000;287: 1433–1438.

19. Johansson CB, Svensson M, Wallstedt L, et al. Neural stem cells in the adult human brain. *Exp Cell Res* 1999;**253:**733–736.

20. Ramberg IL, Wasserman D. Prevalence of reported suicidal behaviour in the general population and mental health-care staff. *Psychol Med* 2000;**30:**1189–1196.

21. Pokorny AD. A scheme for classifying suicidal behaviors. In: Beck AT, Resnick HLP, Lettieri DJ (eds). The prediction of suicide. Bowie, Maryland, USA: Charles Press; 1974:29–44.

22. Paykel ES, Myers JJ, Lindenthal JJ, Tanner J. Suicidal feelings in the general population: a prevalence study. *Br J Psychiatry* 1974;**124:**460–469.

23. Beskow J. Suicide and mental disorder in Swedish men. *Acta Psychiatr Scand* 1979;**Suppl 277:** 1–138.

24. Farberow NL, Shneidman ES. The cry for help. New York: McGraw-Hill; 1961.

25. Wolk-Wasserman D. Suicidal communication of persons attempting suicide and responses of significant others. *Acta Psychiatr Scand* 1986;**73:**481–499.

26. Rutter M. Resilience in the face of adversity. Protective factors and resistance to psychiatric disorder. *Br J Psychiatry* 1985;**147:** 598–611.

3
Neurobiology of suicide and attempted suicide

J John Mann and Victoria Arango

Introduction

Suicide is invariably a complication of psychiatric disorders. Psychological autopsies have generally shown that over 90% of people who commit suicide have an identifiable major psychiatric disorder.[1] However, the majority of people with psychiatric disorders never attempt suicide, with the possible exception of those with borderline personality disorder. Mood disorders account for most suicides and are associated with approximately 60% of all cases. Bipolar disorder has a lifetime rate of suicide of 20% and 15% of people with unipolar or major depressive disorder commit suicide. Despite the high lifetime rate of suicide, most people with mood disorders never attempt suicide. This raises the question as to why some people with psychiatric disorders are at risk of suicide and others are not. We have proposed that there is a diathesis, or predisposition, to suicidal behavior. In discussing the biology of suicidal behavior, it is important to distinguish the biological correlates of this diathesis for suicidal behavior, from the biological correlates of the stressors for suicidal behavior such as the primary psychiatric disorder.[1] Each of these two domains has different biological correlates.

There is a lot of evidence that the commonest stressor or trigger of suicide, major depression, is associated with impaired serotonergic function that involves different brain regions but is independent of the serotonergic abnormality associated with the vulnerability or diathesis for suicidal behavior. In major depression there are fewer platelet serotonin transporters,[2] lower levels of 5-hydroxylindoleacetic acid (5-HIAA) in the cerebrospinal fluid (CSF)[3] and a blunted prolactin response to oral fenfluramine[4] and to intravenous L-tryptophan.[5] The antidepressant efficacy of selective serotonin reuptake inhibitors also suggests that there is a deficiency in serotonergic function. The abnormality in serotonergic function in major depression may be a biochemical trait because it is present even when the patient is clinically better.[6]

Evidence that there are biological factors that contribute to the risk of suicidal behavior

There is a considerable body of evidence indicating that suicidal behavior is influenced by familial and genetic factors.[7] The rate of suicide and suicide attempts is higher in the families of suicide attempters than in families of psychiatric controls (patients with the same psychiatric illness or history). Monozygotic twins have a higher rate of concordance for suicide.[7] Roy et al. also found a higher rate of concordance for suicide attempts in monozygotic twins than in dizygotic twins who survived the co-twin's suicide. The largest published twin study found that the concordance rate for a serious suicide attempt in monozygotic twins (23.1%) was more than 17-fold greater than the risk in the total sample. The rate of concordance for attempted suicide was higher than for completed suicide, indicating that both attempted and completed suicide are heritable. Adoption studies have shown that the risk of suicide is transmitted from the biological family to the adoptees at birth, independent of the transmission of mood or psychotic disorders which, is powerful evidence for genetic transmission. Familial studies have shown that the transmission of suicidal behavior is independent of the transmission of psychopathology associated with suicidal behavior. In other words, the familial transmission of the stressors, such as psychiatric illnesses, is independent of the familial transmission of the diathesis for suicidal behavior. This cumulative body of evidence indicates that there are familial, and almost certainly genetic, factors related to the diathesis for suicidal behavior. The consequence of such genetic factors must be a biological abnormality or phenotype.

Biological correlates of attempted suicide

One of the strongest findings in biological psychiatry is the observation that low levels of 5-HIAA in the CSF are associated with a history of serious suicide attempts in patients with mood disorders, schizophrenia or personality disorders.[3] Moreover, it has been shown that low levels of 5-HIAA in the CSF can predict future suicide and suicide attempts. Studies of CSF 5-HIAA levels in humans and in non-human primates indicate that this index of serotonergic activity in the brain is a biochemical trait that is under significant genetic control. As a biochemical trait under genetic control, it may be one mechanism by which genes can influence behavior, and specifically by which genes can influence the risk for suicidal behavior. Since this marker of serotonin function is low in relationship to suicidal behavior in a variety of psychiatric illnesses, it is not merely a marker of these various psychiatric illnesses, but a biological index of the vulnerability to suicidal behavior associated with these illnesses. We have shown that the more lethal the suicidal behavior, the lower the level of 5-HIAA in the CSF. 5-HIAA is the major breakdown product of serotonin and is proportional to the degree of serotonergic activity in the brain. Some other indices of serotonergic function also include hormone responses to the release of serotonin, such as the prolactin level after the administration of the fenfluramine, a serotonin-releasing agent. Furthermore, platelets have many functions that are mediated by serotonin and provide an easily accessible measure of serotonin function, albeit not in the brain. Both platelet measures and prolactin responses to fenfluramine are indicative of abnormalities in the serotonin system in those who have made suicide attempts compared with psychiatric controls, and the alteration in these serotonin indices is proportional to the seriousness of the suicide attempt in terms of the degree of physical (as opposed to psychological) harm inflicted.

Genetic correlates of neurobiology and suicidal behavior

One approach to determining which genes mediate the risk of suicidal behavior is to examine so-called candidate genes. Candidate genes are most commonly identified because they are involved with neurobiological systems that are already known to be abnormal and to contribute to the pathology of the condition of interest (in this case suicidal behavior). As noted above, the serotonergic system is abnormal in suicide attempters and it appears to represent part of the biology of the diathesis or the vulnerability for suicidal behavior.

One candidate gene that has received particular attention is the gene for tryptophan hydroxylase, which is the enzyme that is involved in the rate-limiting step in the synthesis of serotonin. An abnormality in the production of serotonin may underlie the reduced serotonergic function that is observed in serious suicide attempters. Several studies have demonstrated an association between a polymorphism in the tryptophan hydroxylase gene in intron 7 and suicidal behavior. Those who make suicide attempts are distinguished from those who have the same psychiatric disorder but do not make suicide attempts by having more of a less frequent variant of this gene (U-allele).[8] In addition, this less common variant is associated with lower levels of 5-HIAA in the CSF and a blunted prolactin response to fenfluramine. In other words, two indices of reduced serotonergic function correlate with this less frequent form of the gene, the same form that has been found in association with suicidal behavior in several studies.

These results are preliminary and need further replication, but they illustrate the potential of this strategy. The ultimate goal of this strategy is both to understand the biological factors that contribute to the risk of suicidal behavior and to develop a blood test that will aid the clinician in detecting higher-risk patients.

Biological correlates of completed suicide

Completed suicide is the most serious form of suicidal behavior and one would therefore predict that it would be associated with the most extreme biological abnormalities in terms of the diathesis. This group of patients is also different from suicide attempters in the sense that the brain may be available for study and biochemical analysis. Thus, studies of completed suicide not only look at the most extreme form of this behavior, but also afford the opportunity to examine brain biochemistry directly instead of using indirect methods, such as CSF, pharmacological challenges or platelets.

Early biological studies demonstrated that there was a reduction in levels of serotonin or its breakdown product, 5-HIAA, in the brain stem of suicide victims.[9] The brain stem contains all of the body's serotoninergic neurons, which then project to the rest of the brain to innervate millions of other cells. Thus, the observation that there may be modest reductions in serotonin or 5-HIAA in the brain stem suggests that these brain stem neurons are less active in suicide victims.

A second important observation made from these studies was that the reduction in 5-HIAA or serotonin was similar in degree in suicide victims regardless of the psychiatric diagnosis. Hence, analogous to the findings with CSF 5-HIAA, the brain stem results suggest that this reduction in serotonergic function in suicide victims is associated with the suicide and not with the psychiatric disorder.[9] This fits with our contention that the reduction in serotonergic function in association with suicidal acts is a correlate of the diathesis, or the vulnerability, for suicidal behavior rather than with the stressor, such as a psychiatric illness. Subsequent studies have mapped neuroreceptor changes throughout the brain of suicide victims and have indicated that these changes are particularly striking in the region of the ventral or orbital prefrontal cortex.

Most studies have found that suicide victims have fewer serotonin transporter sites. We have reported that this finding is most striking in the ventral or orbital prefrontal cortex. Many studies, but not all, have found an increase in prefrontal cortical serotonin-5HT$_1$A receptor binding in the brain of suicide victims. Moreover, the binding of platelets to serotonin-5HT$_1$A receptors also appears to be increased in suicidal patients. This possible systemic effect raises the possibility of a genetic mechanism. Although membrane binding studies have generated conflicting results, autoradiographic studies of serotonin-5HT$_2$A binding in suicide victims reported increased binding. Moreover, one study has reported that the increase in serotonin-5HT$_2$A binding is localized to the orbital prefrontal cortex.[10] This ventral area of the prefrontal cortex has been shown in other studies to be involved in behavioral inhibition. Damage to this area of the brain results in disinhibitory behaviors and, potentially, an increased risk of suicide and aggressive behaviors.

We have therefore postulated that serotonergic input to this area of the brain is involved in behavioral inhibition, and that impairment of this input or damage to this area of the brain results in behavioral disinhibition, thereby increasing the likelihood that an affected person will act on powerful emotions or thoughts or feelings, such as suicidal ideation. The importance of this suggestion is that evaluating this area of the brain using brain imaging techniques that are currently in development may offer the clinician another way of testing patients to evaluate the possibility of a vulnerability or predisposition to suicidal behavior.

The role of aggression and impulsivity in suicide risk

It has now been demonstrated by several studies that those who attempt suicide have an increased severity of life-time aggressive and impulsive behaviors.[11] These behavioral traits reflect a fundamental predisposition to act on powerful feelings that may be due to an impairment of serotonin input into the ventral prefrontal cortex, as discussed above.[1] It is therefore noteworthy that studies of pathologically aggressive patients and of aggression in nonhuman primates and other species have demonstrated an association with low serotonergic activity. Thus, low serotonergic activity is not only related to the predisposition to suicidal behavior but also to the predisposition to aggressive and impulsive behaviors in general. Significant aggressive behavior also has a genetic component, and it may be that there is a genetic element common to both suicidal behavior and aggressive behavior. This remains a subject for future research.

Conclusion

The study of the biology of suicidal behavior has provided considerable insights into mechanisms of risk for this behavior and potential future laboratory tests that may aid the clinician in evaluating suicide risk.

References

1. Mann JJ. The neurobiology of suicide. *Nature Med* 1998;**4:**25–30.

2. Owens MJ, Nemeroff CB. Role of serotonin in the pathophysiology of depression: focus on the serotonin transporter. *Clin Chem* 1994;**40:**288–295.

3. Åsberg M. Neurotransmitters and suicidal behavior. The evidence from cerebrospinal fluid studies. *Ann N Y Acad Sci* 1997;**836:** 158–181.

4. O'Keane V, Dinan TG. Prolactin and cortisol responses to D-fenfluramine in major depression: evidence for diminished responsivity of central serotonergic function. *Am J Psychiatry* 1991;**148:** 1009–1015.

5. Delgado PL, Charney DS, Price

LH, et al. Serotonin function and the mechanism of antidepressant action. Reversal of antidepressant-induced remission by rapid depletion of plasma tryptophan. *Arch Gen Psychiatry* 1990;**47:**411–418.

6. Flory JD, Mann JJ, Manuck SB, Muldoon MF. Recovery from major depression is not associated with normalization of serotonergic function. *Biol Psychiatry* 1998;**43:**320–326.

7. Roy A, Rylander G, Sarchiapone M. Genetics of suicide. Family studies and molecular genetics. *Ann N Y Acad Sci* 1997;**836:** 135–157.

8. Mann JJ, Malone KM, Nielsen DA, et al. Possible association of a polymorphism of the tryptophan hydroxylase gene with suicidal behavior in depressed patients. *Am J Psychiatry* 1997;**154:** 1451–1453.

9. Arango V, Underwood MD, Mann JJ. Biologic alterations in the brainstem of suicides. *Psychiatr Clin North Am* 1997;**20:**581–593.

10. Kassir SA, Underwood MD, Bakalian MJ, et al. 5-HT1A binding in dorsal and median raphe nuclei of suicide victims. *Soc Neurosci Abstr* 1998;**24:**1274.

11. Mann JJ, Waternaux C, Haas GL, Malone KM. Towards a clinical model of suicidal behavior in psychiatric patients. *Am J Psychiatry* 1999;**156:**181–189.

Section III
Risk groups for suicide

IIIA Psychiatric disorders
IIIB Personality disorders
IIIC Somatic disorders
IIID Social conditions

IIIA
Psychiatric disorders

4
Affective disorders and suicide

Danuta Wasserman

Introduction

Affective disorder, especially depression, is the single psychiatric diagnosis most strongly linked with suicide. Most patients who commit suicide show several symptoms of depression, and up to 60% have fully diagnosable affective disorder. In older follow-up studies of different groups of depressed patients, lifetime suicide mortality from major depressive disorder seem to be overestimated. In more recent studies, the estimated rate is 10–15%.[1,2] The risk of suicide varies between the subtypes of depression.[3,4]

The overwhelming majority of depressed patients do not take their own lives. Depression is, after all, a very common illness: its estimated prevalence (the proportion of people who have depression at that point in time) is 3–5%,[5] and the lifetime prevalence is approximately 22–24% for women and 15–16% for men. However, it is important to remember that suicide risk is high in untreated patients with depression, especially if comorbidity and negative life events are present.[6,7]

Major depressive disorder

In depression, the central experience is despondency, with marked feelings of emptiness, indifference and hopelessness.[8] Symptoms vary in different age groups and between the sexes.[9–11] Older depressed people very often show signs of restlessness, have difficulty in sitting still and have more somatic symptoms. Their medication can obscure the mental symptoms and make depression more difficult to diagnose. Among middle age men, depression may sometimes be manifested by irritability, awkwardness in interpersonal relations, touchiness, sensitivity to criticism, aggression and even fits of rage. Adolescents quite frequently take refuge in sleep, shutting out the outside world. Diagnosing depression in the young is often complicated owing to the interplay with normal developmental stages. The first striking sign of depression may be a deterioration in school grades, with concentration difficulties that are perceived as laziness and truancy. Feelings of failure and hopelessness are marked. Depressed adolescents' diurnal rhythm may tend to be reversed, and anxiety may sometimes drive them to seek consolation in food. In other cases, they lose weight sharply. Anorexia nervosa or bulimia often coincide with depression in the young (see Chapter 7). For boys, depression is often associated with behavioural disturbances: they may become rowdy, aggressive and highly irritable, and they may resort to violence. Comorbidity in the form of abuse of cannabis, other drugs and alcohol is common.

Anhedonia, concentration difficulties, anxiety and alcohol abuse appear to be short-term predictors of suicide and attempted suicide, while mood fluctuations and feelings of hopelessness are long-term predictors.[12]

Melancholia

Self-belittlement, an exaggerated sense of guilt, a feeling that life is pointless and that one has failed in everything are very often accompanied by severe recurrent suicidal thoughts and thoughts about death. However, the risk of suicide usually first becomes prominent when the patient is in the process of improvement and the psychomotoric inhibition decreases while, at the same time, expectations about the capacity to cope with the psychosocial situation are still very negative. For some patients, confrontation with the reality is experienced as being so frightful and filled with anguish that suicide may appear to be the only solution.

Psychotic depression with delusions or hallucinations has been found to be relatively rare among people who commit suicide.

Male depression

It is not unusual for men to refrain from seeking professional help even when they are severely depressed. When they finally see a doctor, their depression often remains unrecognized and thus untreated. It is not deemed compatible with the male role to be weak, to cry or to be depressed. This may contribute to the fact that men deny their depression and are disinclined to speak of their despondency. It is hardly surprising that depression in men often centres on their occupation and workplace. Becoming unemployed means losing not only the job and income, but also colleagues, fellowship and the structure for life's daily routines. Loss of status is often harder for men to bear than for women, who base their identity to a much larger extent on their families, children and friends.

Men who become depressed develop different symptoms from

women. The depressed man seldom refers to his anxiety, sorrow or despondency. His depression is manifested in poor performance at work, at home or in his leisure activities. Quite frequently, he compensates with intense and non-productive activity. Restlessness, irritability, quarrelsomeness and lack of concentration are typical components. Men probably succumb to depression to a far higher degree than the statistics suggest, but their depression is concealed by alcohol consumption, increased aggressiveness, violence and suicide.[13]

An untreated depression may become so serious that suicide seems the only way out for a man who has difficulty in confiding in anyone and in seeking medical help. Since depressed men very seldom seek psychiatric help, male depression should be brought to the attention of general practitioners, company doctors and other somatic physicians (see Chapter 25). It is recommended that, for men, treatment should be commenced without all the criteria for major depression being fulfilled.

Masked depression

In suicidal patients, it is not unusual for depression to be masked by painful conditions or physical symptoms other than pain, without any underlying physical illness or organ injury. Patients with symptoms of this kind often have difficulty in expressing themselves, in verbalizing their psychological problems and in describing their life situation. The bodily symptoms are a form of communication, signalling that something is wrong, and these symptoms may be a reaction to a life situation that the patient finds unbearable. Having a physical illness is more accepted, not only in Western culture but elsewhere as well. People's inability to get in touch with their own experience can be reinforced by cultures in which mental illness is the object of prejudice.

In suicidal people with masked depression, symptoms may take the form of aches and pains localized to joints, muscles and other parts of the body, but also tiredness, chronic fatigue, dizziness, numbness in the arms and legs or a feeling of pressure in the head. It is for these symptoms that these patients consult their doctor. A systematic review of the suicidal patient's life situation often reveals severe conflicts in the family or at work and marked suicidal ideation. General practitioners should be trained to detect masked depression, suicidal thoughts and various types of suicidal communication so as to be able to prevent suicide attempts and suicide.

Dysthymia

The course of dysthymia is less periodical than that of major depressive disorder. People with dysthymia experience a state of depression that is more or less constant but somewhat mild as compared to major depression. Many dysthymic states start in childhood and are widely regarded as personality disorders with gloom as the keynote; others see them as anxiety disorders. The psychological development of people with dysthymia is often inhibited, since they find it difficult to believe in their own abilities and a bright future for themselves.

Suicide risk in dysthymia may be comparable to that in most severe forms of affective disorders, although the relative importance of the roles played in suicidality by the actual depression, the anxiety component or comorbidity in the form of personality disorder is impossible to ascertain.

Not infrequently, a suicidal patient may have double depression, with major depressive disorder on top of dysthymia.

Bipolar states and mania

There is some difference in lifetime suicide risk between patients with unipolar major affective disorder (15%) and those with bipolar major affective disorder (20%).[13,14]

The majority of patients with a bipolar illness who commit suicide are, at the time of death, in the throes of a major depressive episode or in a mixed depressive state.[15] Suicide during the manic phase is relatively rare. Hypomanic and manic states are often followed by profound depression, with remorse and a conviction that one has messed up one's life during the manic period. This may, in certain cases, be a contributory factor in suicide. Suicide rates appear to be the same among patients with illnesses of bipolar 1 and bipolar 2 type. 'Bipolar 1' means a disorder in which mania has occurred on at least one occasion; 'bipolar 2' refers to a disorder where hypomania has occurred but mania has not. However, it is possible that bipolar 2 illness is not recognised owing to the low reliability of the hypomania diagnosis.

Degrees of suicidality appear to be equal for men and women suffering from bipolar illnesses, but men's suicides take place earlier in the course of the illness than women's. However, one should not ignore observations that serious suicide attempts and suicides can also take place late in the course of affective illness.

Comorbidity

Concurrent depression and anxiety that seem to be aetiologically related and are difficult to separate are typical of suicidal patients.[16]

People with major depressive disorder who commit suicide also often show comorbidity of alcohol and other substance misuse, multiple physical diseases and various personality disorders. Comorbidity varies according to sex and age. Older patients have more somatic illnesses than younger ones, while young patients often exhibit various types of personality disorder and men engage in psychoactive substance abuse. Depressive symptoms are also frequently present in schizophrenic patients who commit suicide. Manic–depressive patients who commit suicide, on the other hand, are often dependent on alcohol.[6]

Medical consultations before suicide

In more than 60% of cases, people who commit suicide consult psychiatrists in the year before the act, and in many cases as late as in the week before the act (see Chapter 26). Women have more contacts with psychiatric care services, while men more frequently consult general practitioners or other doctors. However, as many as 20% of patients have no medical consultations before committing suicide.

Doctors do not always think of suicide risk, since many of the patients they have seen have, before suicide, shown clear calming or masked depression. 'Clear calming' means that suicidal individuals are not anxiety driven because they decided to take their own life and also which method of suicide to use. Male patients seldom spontaneously communicate their suicidal intentions and many of them show signs of masked depression, making it difficult for a correct psychiatric diagnosis.

Antidepressants as means of committing suicide

Apprehension is often expressed about the elevated risk of suicide and attempted suicide associated with the treatment of depression with antidepressant drugs. The danger that certain antidepressants are more toxic than others and may, in the event of an overdose, have severe consequences and even be lethal should not, of course, be underestimated. Approximately 5–8% of people who take their own lives use antidepressants as a means of intoxication.[17] Accordingly, the great majority of depressed people who die from suicide use a method other than poisoning with antidepressants. However, the antidepressants received during a previous treatment or antidepressants obtained from relatives can be used as a means of suicide.

The older tricyclic antidepressants have relatively high overdose toxicity; the newer antidepressants are less toxic. But, even the newer agents can be used for self-destructive purposes. What counts here, obviously, is not only the properties of the tablets ingested but also the patient's intention, as expressed in the quantity of tablets swallowed.

Doctors and relatives alike should bear in mind that there is a risk of suicidal acts at the commencement of treatment with antidepressants before the full effect is achieved,[18] since patients' symptoms improve after approximately 2–3 weeks' treatment and their psychomotor inhibitions relax while their perceptions of the illness and (very often) poor psychosocial situation still persist. Moreover, one should be mindful of the fact that anxiety, which is a powerful impetus towards suicidal acts, is intensified at the beginning of treatment with certain antidepressants. Active follow-up with face-to-face supportive discussions is therefore important.

Treatment of depression and prevention of suicide

Although assessing the suicide preventive effects of various treatments is subject to several methodological difficulties (partly because of the divergent selection factors used in different studies, and partly because of information bias and random fluctuations in suicide rates in small populations), the results of existing studies and clinical experience are clearly promising (see Chapters 19, 20, 24 and 25). Both psychotherapeutical and pharmacological treatments have good effects.

Unfortunately, although some 60% of people seek help shortly before committing suicide, only about 15% receive antidepressant prescriptions and, of these, half show poor compliance and discontinue their medication 2–3 weeks before the suicide. For others, the dosage is often insufficient. According to studies from Sweden and Finland, only 3–6% of those who died from suicide were receiving adequate dosages of antidepressant medication.[13,17] Psychotherapeutic treatment was also very seldom available. Electroconvulsive therapy and treatment with lithium were uncommon. According to a Finnish study, only 3% of people who died from suicide had received electroconvulsive therapy and 3% had received lithium treatment.[13]

Effective treatment of depression with both pharmacological and psychological methods is the foremost strategy of suicide prevention among young people, the middle-aged and the elderly alike. Treatment of depression appears, however, to be of more benefit in preventing suicide in women than in men.

Case history:
Keeping problems to oneself

Jussi, aged 40

Jussi, a 40-year-old Finnish-born factory worker, had moved to Sweden several years ago in search of a better job. He was engaged to, and lived with, a Finnish woman who was 1 year his senior and with whom he was expecting a child. The woman's four children from a previous marriage were in their father's care. Jussi was described as taciturn, placid, reliable, helpful and concerned about his family. Married once previously, he had a child from the marriage, who was looked after by his ex-wife.

In the past 6 months his duties at the factory had changed and he no longer enjoyed his job. Although he had not striven to keep his ordinary duties, he felt hurt and disappointed when a colleague was chosen to replace him.

Over the past months, his private life had also changed. He had stopped seeing his siblings, who also lived in Sweden, and he refused to visit his parents in Finland although they had warmly invited him, his fiancée and her children to a big family gathering.

From time to time he complained of pain in the same part of his back that he had strained while renovating a boat.

In the past 4 weeks, Jussi had begun losing interest in everything. Even painting his beloved boat did not appeal to him, although the sailing trips of the spring and summer were approaching. He could be deeply despondent one moment and irritable and restless the next. Previously very even-tempered, he had on one occasion hit his fiancée's 5-year-old son, who was briefly visiting them. This was the impetus for his fiancée's suggestion that Jussi should see a doctor.

Jussi went to see his general practitioner. During the consultation he was reserved and obviously unaccustomed to talking about his situation at work and in his private life. He did not tell the doctor that he felt very lonely and under pressure because of his fiancée's pregnancy, nor did he refer to his worry about how they would cope financially, having to support not only the child from his first marriage but also the baby they were expecting and his fiancée's other children. He shared neither with the doctor nor with anyone else his intensive brooding about what kind of mother his fiancée would turn out to be, since she had not looked after her own children from her previous relationship.

Jussi also omitted to tell the doctor that everything had felt black and difficult over the past month. The idea of hanging himself kept coming back to him. A colleague had taken his own life 1 year before and his maternal grandfather, who had been depressed, had hanged himself when Jussi was a child. These ideas were not conveyed to the doctor, who prescribed a painkiller.

The prescription did not help, and the family sensed Jussi's growing dependency and inactivity. Besides backache, he began getting headaches and stomach aches, and his eating habits deteriorated. In 3 weeks, he lost several kilograms in weight. Jussi became more and more detached from his family. He began resorting to alcohol to get to sleep. No longer interested in anything, he became passive, withdrawn and sluggish.

One day he refused to see an assistant from the Finnish housing agency whom he and his fiancée had an appointment with to hear about opportunities for getting a better flat. In despair his fiancée turned to the

Finnish church, and the parson promised to visit them at home. Jussi always felt uneasy in the presence of the parson, whom he feared and considered stern.

On the day before the parson's visit, Jussi went out early in the morning in the garden and hanged himself. He was found by a passing factory guard and cut down. After resuscitation, he was admitted to a psychiatric unit. After his suicide attempt, Jussi was treated with electroconvulsive therapy, followed by antidepressants, and underwent family therapy with his fiancée.

References

1. Blair-West GW, Mellsop GW, Eyeson-Annan ML. Down-rating lifetime suicide risk in major depression. *Acta Psychiatr Scand* 1997;**95**:259–263.

2. Wulsin LR, Vaillant GE, Wells VE. A systematic review of the mortality of depression. *Psychosomatic Medicine* 1999;**61**:6–17.

3. Buchholtz-Hansen P, Wang A, Kragh-Sörensen P. Mortality in major affective disorder: relationship to subtype of depression. The Danish University Antidepressant Group. *Acta Psychiatr Scand* 1993;**87**:329–335.

4. Rihmer Z, Barsi J, Arato M, Demeter E. Suicide in subtypes of primary major depression. *J Affective Disord* 1990;**18**:221–225.

5. Kessler R, McGonagle KA, Zhao S, et al. Lifetime and 12-month prevalence of DSM-III-R psychiatric disorders in the United States. *Arch Gen Psychiatry* 1994;**51**:8–19.

6. Henriksson M, Aro H, Marttunen M, et al. Mental disorders and comorbidity in suicide. *Am J Psychiatry* 1993;**150**:935–940.

7. Regier D, Burke J, Burke K. Comorbidity of affective and anxiety disorders in the NIMH Epidemiologic Catchment Area Program. In: Maser J, Cloninger R (eds). Comorbidity of mood and anxiety disorders. Washington, DC, USA: American Psychiatric Press; 1990:113–122.

8. Modestin J, Kopp W. Study on suicide in depressed inpatients. *J Affective Disord* 1988;**15**:157–162.

9. Blumenthal SJ. An overview and synopsis of risk factors, assessment, and treatment of suicidal patients over the life cycle. In: Blumenthal SJ, Kupfer DI (eds). Suicide over the life cycle: risk factors, assessment, and treatment of suicidal patients. Washington, DC, USA: American Psychiatric Press; 1990:685–733.

10. Conwell Y, Duberstein PR, Cox C, et al. Relationships of age and axis I diagnoses in victims of completed suicide: a psychological autopsy study. *Am J Psychiatry* 1996;**153**:1001–1008.

11. Kendler K, Kessler R, Neale M, et al. The prediction of major depression in women: toward an integrated etiologic model. *Am J Psychiatry* 1993; **150**:1139–1148.

12. Fawcett J, Scheftner W, Fogg L, et al. Time-related predictors of suicide in major affective disorder. *Am J Psychiatry* 1990;**147**:1189–1194.

13. Isometsä E, Lönnqvist J. Suicide in

mood disorders. In: Botsis JA, Soldatos CR, Stefanis CN (eds). Suicide: biopsychosocial approaches. Amsterdam, The Netherlands: Elsevier; 1997:33–47.

14. Lester D. Suicidal behavior in bipolar and unipolar affective disorders: a meta-analysis. *J Affective Disord* 1993;**27:**117–121.

15. Simpson SG, Jamison KR. The risk of suicide in patients with bipolar disorders. *J Clin Psychiatry* 1999;**60(Suppl 2):**53–56.

16. Allgulander C. Suicide and mortality patterns in anxiety neurosis and depressive neurosis. *Arch Gen Psychiatry* 1994;**51:**708–712.

17. Isacsson G, Holmgren P, Wasserman D, Bergman U. Use of antidepressants among people committing suicide in Sweden. *BMJ* 1994;**308:**506–509.

18. Schweizer E, Dever A, Clary C. Suicide upon recovery from depression: a clinical note. *J Nerv Ment Dis* 1988;**176:**633–636.

5
Alcoholism, other psychoactive substance misuse and suicide

Danuta Wasserman

Introduction

The term 'alcohol and other psychoactive substance misuse' covers states from problematic use to established abuse and dependence. The validity of a diagnosis of dependence on alcohol or another psychoactive substance is good in contrast to the validity of a diagnosis of abuse or high consumption due to existing disagreement about definitions.

Adults in the West consume alcohol in everyday social situations. Some drink to reduce stress or to relieve their inhibitions and anxiety on social occasions because it helps to embolden them in their contacts with others. However, excessive alcohol consumption has devastating consequences in the long term.

Definition of high consumption of alcohol

Since the role of alcohol varies from one setting and culture to another, the level defined as 'high' and deemed to pose risks of developing somatic or psychiatric complications differs from one country to the next and between men and women. In the UK and Sweden, a man who drinks more than 210 g (equivalent to three and a half bottles of wine) and a woman who drinks more than 140 g of ethanol (equivalent to two and a half bottles of wine) per week is assigned to the high-consumption group. The limits are higher in Finland and lower in the USA.

Alcohol abuse and alcohol dependence

Figures for alcohol abuse and dependence vary between countries and between social and ethnic groups. In the National Comorbidity Survey from the USA,[1] lifetime prevalence of alcohol dependence is estimated at 20% and alcohol abuse at around 12% for men. The corresponding figures for women are roughly 8% and 6%, respectively. The state of dependence does not need to be lifelong.

49

Drug abuse and dependence

In the above-mentioned National Comorbidity Survey, drug dependence is estimated at around 9% and drug abuse at some 5% for men. The corresponding figures for women are 6% and 3%, respectively. Drug misusers often use a mixture of alcohol and prescription drugs. Reliable data on the rates of abuse and of dependence on illicit drugs in different countries are lacking. In some countries, up to 30% of middle-aged and elderly adults are estimated to have taken illicit drugs at some time in their lives.[2]

Suicide risk

For people who are dependent on alcohol, mortality is four times that of the population as a whole, and half of these deaths have violent causes, especially suicide. Longitudinal follow-up studies of alcohol-dependent patients show that approximately 7% die from suicide.[3] The suicide mortality rate of drug abusers is estimated to be at the same level as that of alcoholics.[4,5] Retrospective studies have shown that alcohol abuse and dependence characterized 15–50% of people who take their own lives, depending on the population surveyed and also on sex and age. Alcohol problems are more often observed in young people and middle-aged men who commit suicide than in other groups. Alcoholism in connection with suicide among women and the elderly is often under-reported, probably owing to shame.[6]

For many people, suicide risk does not necessarily occur as a result of severe dependence.[7] For many, occasions of high consumption or drunkenness can also entail risks of accidents, violence and suicide when their ability to curb impulses to act, as well as their capacity for constructive thought, is impaired. The alcohol causes a deterioration in cognitive capacity and, accordingly, in flexibility and the ability to find alternative solutions. Suicidal alcohol misusers are often characterized by a fairly good psychosocial coping ability. Their suicides take place when they are in a drunken state and numerous problems have accumulated. Good psychosocial functioning may perhaps explain why alcoholics who eventually take their own lives receive so little psychiatric treatment.

A Finnish study[8] has shown that alcohol abusers who died from suicide and who were employed had taken their own lives at weekends to a significantly higher extent than unemployed alcohol abusers. People with a tendency towards anxiety and depression are at high risk of suicide when the effect of alcohol wears off, since these symptoms are exacerbated in conjunction with a hangover.

Suicidal process

Suicidal substance misusers very often use direct, verbal suicidal communication immediately before the suicidal act, but also long before it. They may, when either intoxicated or sober, accuse members of their immediate family of causing their difficulties and, by implication, their suicidal crises. These accusations are not infrequently expressed during quarrels and in tumultuous circumstances. The purpose of this type of communication may, paradoxically enough, be to satisfy their needs for attention and for support from their nearest family members. The suicidal process is usually prolonged in substance misusers, lasting many years.

Unfortunately, suicidal substance misusers experience many negative reactions to their suicidal communication from both relatives and healthcare staff, who may respond with marked ambivalence and aggressiveness, thereby accelerating the development of the suicidal process towards suicide.

Losing a vitally important relationship is often the immediate factor that precipitates suicide. A suicidal substance misuser then loses not only love, but also part of his or her already weak self-esteem, since the person who has been lost has often performed the function not only of providing support but also of bolstering the misuser's self-esteem. The more dependence that misusers experience in their relationships, the greater the risk that separation may push them into chaos, regression and self-destructive acts.[9] Hypersensitivity to separations among substance misusers is rooted in their previous lives. They have often lacked support in the parental home and had no one to talk to. Early separations due to death, divorce in the family of origin or a move away from home, as well as social deprivation and parents' alcoholism and, quite frequently, mental illness, contribute to the lack of good identification objects. This impedes development of strong self-esteem and adequate coping strategies. Troubled relationships later in adult life, with the threat of impending separation, often show repetition of previous patterns and activate earlier feelings of impotence, hopelessness and rage. It may then be only a short step to a point at which suicidal behaviour presents itself as the only way out.

Suicidal substance misusers are also highly sensitive, easily offended and inclined to interpret everything in negative terms. It is not unusual for them to provoke negative reactions from others, consciously or unconsciously, by their manner and behaviour, and this in turn may result in them feeling rejected, unwanted and excluded. A vicious circle, with a sense of hopelessness and risk of suicidal behaviour, may easily arise.

When life feels pointless and cheerless, suicidal thoughts and a longing for death may arise even in people who are normally far from suicidality. For most people, however, the step from a suicidal thought to a suicidal act is a long one. In substance misusers, when their judgement is blunted and impulses are freed from inhibition, the step from thought to act is short. This is why, to a far greater extent than in other people, losses, separations and various types of offence that would be perceived by others to be insignificant may be the factors precipitating suicide in substance misusers (see also Chapters 2 and 13).

Comorbidity

Estimating the importance of alcohol or other psychoactive substance misuse as a single factor in suicide is difficult, since substance misusers very often have comorbidity of affective disorders, anxiety disorders and personality disorders, especially of the borderline type.[8–12]

Alcoholism is, however, thought to rank second, after affective disorder, as a risk factor for suicide. Affective disorders are common in alcoholics of both sexes. In women, the onset of major depressive disorder precedes the alcohol dependence in two-thirds of cases. In men, on the other hand, alcohol abuse or dependence precede affective disorders in almost 80% of cases.

Many alcoholics who die from suicide suffer from deep depressions that are quite frequently protracted, with a mean length of year 1; unfortunately, they show atypical symptoms, which makes detection difficult. Another factor that sometimes impedes diagnosis of depression in suicidal alcoholics is that their personality disorders mask their depression symptoms.[6]

Teenage alcoholics who die from suicide are often characterized by severe and protracted psychiatric morbidity, psychosocial dysfunction and antisocial behaviour.[13] The same often applies to their families. In some countries such as the Nordic countries, in contrast to others such as the USA, the prevalence of alcoholism and substance abuse among adolescent female suicides is as high as it is among the adolescent males. Young heavy drinkers typically drink at weekends, and this pattern is reflected in the fact that suicides are clustered around weekends.[8]

Diagnosis and treatment

The American Psychiatric Association (1995) has summarized the results from various surveys, and reported several forms of beneficial therapy.[14] The duration of treatment may vary, but to bring about changes in moderate alcohol dependence it should not be less than 6 months. Treatment commonly lasts up to 2 years. It is important to maintain patient contact even if benefits are attained initially. When there is a risk of suicidal behaviour, detoxification should take place on an inpatient basis and for a sufficiently long period.

Suicidal male alcoholics often consult general practitioners or emergency somatic departments for physical ailments. It is sometimes difficult for general practitioners to detect alcoholism and substance misuse if the patient is reticent. Structured forms, such as the CAGE questionnaire,[15] may then be helpful. 'CAGE' stands for Cut down, Annoyance, Guilty feelings, Eye opener. The CAGE acronym refers to the four questions: Have you ever felt you should *Cut down* on your drinking? Have people *Annoyed* you by criticizing your drinking? Have you every felt bad or *Guilty* about your drinking? And have you ever had a drink first thing in the morning to steady your nerves or to get rid of a hangover (*Eye opener*)?

In dealing with suicidal male alcoholics a time-line follow-back technique, involving a systematic review of the past 3 months' alcohol and drug consumption in terms of both pattern and quantity, is another possibility. Abuse and dependence is often unrecognized in female misusers (even though many of them are psychiatric patients), owing to women's unwillingness to admit their alcohol habits and doctors' lack of alertness.

Treatment must take into consideration the type and degree of misuse, the somatic status, psychiatric comorbidity, the level of social functioning and problems in the spheres of life that are affected by the misuse. Measures may range from simple provision of advice or intervention to inpatient care, especially if there is an acute suicide risk.

Psychosocial support

In choosing psychological treatment, personality factors must be taken into account. The treatment objectives should be defined in operational terms, preferably in writing, and followed up regularly. Many suicidal alcoholics and drug misusers have proved to be cognitively more concrete than abstract. It therefore seems important to link the patient's mental phenomena with highly concrete objectives on a rising scale of difficulty. Relatives should be involved in the treatment process, in view of the negative emotional climate in the family that often characterizes suicidal substance misusers.[14]

Psychotherapy

Alcoholics and drug misusers often swing between overrating and disparaging themselves and other people – health-care staff included, and they have a tendency to take offence and easily feel hurt and rejected, which can result in a negative attitude to treatment and poor compliance. Moreover, suicidal misusers' impulsiveness and sense that 'it's now or never' mean that psychological and medical treatment needs to be flexible and adjusted to the psychological needs of the patient.[9,14]

Psychotherapeutic treatments include group, family and individual therapy. For adolescents, family therapy is recommended. Cognitive psychotherapy and psychoeducative techniques, in which specific treatment objectives are defined for both the short and the long term, have proved successful.[14]

Medication

Before an alcoholic is diagnosed as suffering from depression, the detoxification process should be completed. In the first few days of 'detox', some 60% of alcoholics show several depressive symptoms. After 2 weeks, only one patient in five shows signs of depression. Alcohol abusers should therefore be sober for at least 2 weeks before their need for antidepressant treatment can be assessed.[16] On the other hand, for alcoholics who have previously been diagnosed as depressed and who are at risk of suicide, antidepressant medication should be commenced earlier.

When alcoholics are treated with antidepressants, not only is their depression relieved but their craving for alcohol diminishes. There are also studies that show that antidepressants can both remedy depression and prevent a relapse into abuse for drug addicts as well. However, pharmacological treatment must always be combined with psychosocial support.

Access to alcohol

Hereditary factors and psychosocial and sociocultural factors play a roughly equal part in causing alcoholism. The easy availability of alcohol and cultural habits that encourage its consumption therefore have a negative bearing on the rate of mortality from suicide (see also Chapter 29).

What should be done?

Pay attention to heavy drinkers in risk situations

When a person suddenly incurs problems in interpersonal relationships, at work or in other contexts and starts drinking at weekends, others should take notice. The same applies to young people who show a pattern of heavy weekend drinking and come from high-risk families and to alcohol and drug misusers in work places.

Improve diagnostics, treatment and organization of care

Detection of substance abuse among female psychiatric patients should be improved, and more attention should also be devoted to psychiatric problems among men who abuse alcohol or drugs and whose psychoso-cial functioning is fairly good. Only a minority of substance misusers who commit suicide receive adequate psychiatric help in the last month of their lives, despite their obvious psychiatric morbidity.

The above facts remain true, although both men and women are often in touch with health-care services and communicate their suicidal intent to the staff before committing suicide. The blame may, perhaps, be laid on organizational factors: in many countries, co-operation between sub-stance-abuse units, general practitioners and psychiatric departments is very poor; and the same applies to co-operation with social-welfare authorities who are responsible for rehabilitation. Setting up special healthcare establishments with expertise in treating dual-diagnosis patients may be one solution.

Case history:
Drug initiation

Ann-Marie, aged 30

Small and slender, Ann-Marie tended to arouse intense caring feelings in others much of the time but periodically she was provocative, dismissive and uncommunicative. Her mother had died of cervical cancer when Ann-Marie was 12. Her brother had started abusing drugs, and 2 years after their mother's death he took his own life by shooting himself. It was Ann-Marie who found his body, and relating the experience still made her quiver with emotion. Her father, 20 years older than her mother and a fisherman by trade, became deeply depressed after his wife's death and his son's suicide, and he isolated himself completely. He was unable to take care of his daughter and took no interest in her schooling, social life or future.

Ann-Marie had evidently undergone repeated periods of depression with a clearly seasonal pattern since her early teens. During these peri-ods, she had experienced intense suicidal ideation and a pressing sense that there was nothing to live for. Because of increasing loss of interest in her studies, she had failed to complete her compulsory 9 years of school-ing. The school psychologist, whom she had met more or less regularly, never diagnosed her depression.

At the age of 16 she had been employed as a nanny, but was dis-missed as soon as the family found out that her boyfriend was a well-known drug addict. He introduced Ann-Marie to drugs and alcohol. She was then in contact with the social welfare office, which first arranged hostel accommodation for her and eventually found her temporary employment as an assistant in various shops. She never enjoyed these jobs, and was increasingly drawn into her 'fiancé's circle of associates and his drug-taking habits. Every time conflicts arose with the boyfriend or his associates, pitch-black, uncontrollable feelings of hopelessness and suicidal thoughts swept over her.

Between the ages of 18 and 20, Ann-Marie had been admitted several times to various services for drug-abuse treatment, but she had always checked out after a brief stay and returned to the gang. Her life was constantly in chaos, with numerous people – from the psychiatric clinic, the social services and the police – involved. Ann-Marie was unable to recall the names of various people who bore some kind of responsibility for her and it was obvious that she had not formed any strong ties with any of these carers, or vice versa. They all saw her as a hopeless case.

At the age of 20, she made four suicide attempts in 6 months. These suicide attempts were triggered by police interrogations that arose because of the involvement of Ann-Marie and her 'fiancé' Olle in drug trafficking and a burglary that he had roped her into while on parole from prison. A triangular drama that she was unable to resolve (involving herself, Olle and a temporary boyfriend she lived with during Olle's imprisonment) was another factor that contributed to her suicide attempts.

After the fourth attempt, when she had taken a large number of sleeping pills and was deeply unconscious for several days, she was treated at an intensive care unit. There she came into contact with a female psychiatric nurse, who identified with Ann-Marie's problems and succeeded in motivating her to undergo a long-term cure at a treatment centre for drug abusers.

After several years of rehabilitation, Ann-Marie continued to have regular sessions with a psychotherapist. Ten years after the treatment, at the age of 30, Ann-Marie was still seeing the therapist a few times a year. She had a job she enjoyed, as an assistant nurse at an old people's home. In her spare time she was committed to her voluntary work, helping to rehabilitate former teenage prostitutes. She was not married but had a steady relationship with a plumber of the same age as herself.

References

1. Kessler RC, Nelson CB, McGonagle KA, et al. The epidemiology of co-occurring addictive and mental disorders. Implications for prevention and service utilisation. *Am J Orthopsychiatry* 1996;**66:**17–31.

2. Gerada C, Ashworth M. ABC of mental health: addiction and dependence—I: illicit drugs. *Br Med J* 1997;**315:**297–300.

3. Inskip HM, Harris C, Barraclough B. Lifetime risk of suicide for affective disorder, alcoholism and schizophrenia. *Br J Psychiatry* 1998;**172:**35–37.

4. Oyefeso A, Ghodse H, Clancy C, Corkery JM. Suicide among drug addicts in the UK. *Br J Psychiatry* 1999;**175:**277–282.

5. Öhberg A, Vuori E, Ojanperä I, Lönnqvist J. Alcohol and drugs in suicides. *Br J Psychiatry* 1996; **169:**75–80.

6. Murphy GE. Suicide in alco-
    holism. New York: Oxford Univer-
    sity Press, 1992.

7. Taylor C, Cooper J, Appleby L. Is
    suicide risk taken seriously in
    heavy drinkers who harm them-
    selves? *Acta Psychiatr Scand*
    1999;**100:**309–311.

8. Pirkola S. Alcohol and other sub-
    stance misuse in suicide: a
    review. *Psychiatria Fennica* 1999;
    30:80–92.

9. Wasserman D. Alcohol and suici-
    dal behaviour. *Nordic J Psychia-
    try* 1993;**47:**265–271.

10. Berglund M, Öjehagen A. The
    influence of alcohol drinking and
    alcohol use disorders on psychi-
    atric disorders and suicidal
    behavior. *Alcohol Clin Exp Res*
    1998;**22(Suppl 7):**333–345.

11. Cornelius JR, Salloum IM, Day
    NL, et al. Patterns of suicidality
    and alcohol use in alcoholics with
    major depression. *Alcohol Clin
    Exp Res* 1996;**20:** 1451–1455.

12. Dinwiddie SH, Reich T, Cloninger
    CR. Psychiatric comorbidity and
    suicidality among intravenous
    drug users. *J Clin Psychiatry*
    1992;**53:**364–369.

13. Bukstein O, Brent D, Perper J, et
    al. Risk factors for completed sui-
    cide among adolescents with a
    lifetime history of substance
    abuse: a case-control study. *Acta
    Psychiatr Scand* 1993;**88:**
    403–408.

14. American Psychiatric Association.
    Practice guideline for the treat-
    ment of patients with substance
    use disorders: alcohol, cocaine
    and opioids. *Am J Psychiatry*
    1995;**152(Suppl 11):**1–59.

15. Mayfield D, McLeod G, Hall P.
    The CAGE questionnaire: valida-
    tion of a new alcoholism screen-
    ing instrument. *Am J Psychiatry*
    1974;**131:**1121–1123.

16. Schuckit MA. Drug and Alcohol
    Abuse: A clinical guide to diagno-
    sis and treatment, 4th edn. New
    York: Plenum Publishing; 1995.

6

The anxiety disorders, anxiety symptoms and suicide

Jan Fawcett

Anxiety disorders

According to the Diagnostic and Statistical Manual of Mental Disorders (DSM) IV, there are several anxiety symptoms that can combine to form more or less distinct clinical anxiety disorders. Important categories include:

- generalized anxiety disorder;
- panic disorder;
- various phobic states; and
- obsessive–compulsive disorder.

Post-traumatic stress syndrome belongs also to this group of psychiatric diseases.

Among the anxiety disorders in DSM IV, panic disorder has been specifically studied and data have been presented that associate this anxiety disorder with increased rates of suicide[1] and suicide attempts.[2] There is disagreement as to whether panic disorder alone is sufficient to increase this risk or whether a major affective disorder must also be present to result in an increased rate of suicide. There is growing recognition of a range anxiety disorders that increase the risk of suicidal behaviours when they are present as a comorbid feature of major affective disorders.[3,4] An overview of the international published experience suggests that the degree of increased suicide risk is related to the severity of the anxiety symptoms, and that anxiety symptoms are sometimes not fully recognized by clinicians in patients with major affective disorders.[5] The suicide risk is higher in patients with both anxiety symptoms and affective disorders in comparison to patients who only suffer from affective disorders without anxiety.[6] The idea that a DSM IV anxiety disorder, such as panic disorder, alone confers an increased risk of suicide was suggested by one study, but this was not confirmed by another; therefore, this is yet to be determined.[2,7] Several studies of increased anxiety as a trait or as acutely comorbidity with affective disorders are showing an increased risk of suicidal behaviours in children, adolescents and adults. This is true for the range of anxiety disorders listed above.

Anxiety symptoms

A series of clinical studies have found that severe anxiety symptoms occurring in the context of clinical depressive disorders may be a significant factor in short-term suicide risk and one that is reversible with treatment.[8] This research together with a review of past studies suggests that classic risk factors for suicide, such as prior attempts and suicidal ideation, while associated with long-term risk, may not always be sufficiently useful in the assessment and intervention in acute suicide risk situations.[8] The implications of these findings point to a need for an increased emphasis on the active elicitation and aggressive treatment of anxiety symptoms in patients with symptoms of clinical depression. Up until now, the types of anxiety associated most strongly with suicidal risk are severe psychic anxiety symptoms (characterized by intense feelings of fear or by ruminative and exaggerated worry, panic attacks) and agitation (characterized by distress expressed through physical movement or vocalizations), as well as angry frustration.[5,6,8,9] Emotional outbursts associated with labile mood and loss of control as well as anxiety expressed through dissociative behaviours in combination with depression, are also suspected manifestations of suicidal risk, although these have been somewhat less specifically measured in studies so far.

Depression and anxiety

It has been suggested that depression and anxiety are caused by the same underlying biological vulnerability although, from the clinical point of view, the major difference is that depression is characterized by inhibition whereas in states of anxiety the patient is usually agitated. Thus, it has been documented that regulation of the important neurotransmitters of the brain – dopamine, noradrenaline (norepinephrine) and serotonin – is affected in states of anxiety. It is also known that reinforcement of gamma-aminobutyric acid activity (which inhibits brain activity and thus allows the brain to rest) by benzodiazepines relieves anxiety symptoms.

Suicide risk and severe anxiety

There is evidence relating to the presence of severe anxiety symptoms as a risk factor in suicides in hospitalized patients or those admitted to an emergency facility. A prospective study comparing the presence and severity of symptoms in in-patients with major depression who committed suicide and those who did not has shown that certain features differentiated significantly between the suicide patients and the survivors in the first year of follow-up:[5,6,8]

- the severity of psychic anxiety;
- the occurrence of panic attacks;
- moderate alcohol abuse;
- global insomnia;
- severe anhedonia; and
- poor concentration.

These features were more frequently present in the suicide patients than in the survivors. This was not the case for prior suicide attempts and suicidal ideation, both of which are considered to be standard 'predictors' of suicide risk. The correlation in this study of suicidal ideation and suicide versus non-suicide reached significance and approached significance for prior suicide attempts only in follow-up years 2–10.[5] Thus, severe anxiety and related symptoms may be more useful acute suicide risk factors than the standard 'predictors', which appear more associated with longer-term suicide risk. One explanation for these findings could be that in most studies anxiety symptoms have not been followed closely enough during the first year after the suicide attempt.

Seventy-nine per cent of in-patients who committed suicide were retrospectively reported to manifest evidence of severe psychic anxiety, severe agitation or both in the week before their suicide.[9] Ninety per cent of patients who were admitted to an emergency facility with suicide attempts that were severe enough to require admission and who were immediately interviewed reported severe anxiety symptoms before the attempt; 80% reported associated panic symptoms.[10]

More studies are certainly needed to replicate the validity and to test the sensitivity and specificity of severe anxiety symptoms as acute risk factors as well as to construct an instrument for assessing specific anxiety symptoms in this regard. Also, the severity levels that might be predictive of acute risk of suicide must be further characterized in order to obtain a more effective standard for the assessment of the high-risk suicidal patient.

Treatment

The above-mentioned data suggest that the recognition and rapid treatment of symptoms of severe anxiety may reduce the acute risk of suicide even before the underlying depression can be effectively treated, because of the rapid onset of anxiolytic medications compared with the delayed therapeutic onset of presently available antidepressant therapies.[8]

It is known that some antidepressant agents may worsen the patient's perception of anxiety during the first few weeks of treatment. This effect is seen especially in patients who suffer from depression with a marked anxiety and who are treated with selective serotonin reuptake inhibitors; it is due to stimulation of serotonin-2 receptors. The combination of increased anxiety and simultaneous relaxation of psychomotor inhibition elevates the risk of self-destructive acts such as suicide attempt and suicide. For this reason there is a need for extra vigilance on the part of doctor and family members during the first weeks of treatment. Supplementary supportive psychotherapy for patients suffering from anxiety is usually helpful.

Indeed, the development of safe, rapidly effective treatments that target psychic anxiety, panic attacks and agitation in depressed patients might well enhance treatment outcomes, reduce relapses and significantly decrease suffering in a large proportion of depressed patients who suffer comorbid anxiety symptoms, irrespective of the presence of high suicide risk.

However, there are at present no studies to demonstrate that treatment that specifically targets the symptoms of anxiety and agitation reduces acute suicide risk. The evidence is still circumstantial and indirect, albeit probably logical. Nevertheless, if the severity of anxiety symptoms in depressed patients are recorded and treated aggressively, it can be assumed that suicides can probably be prevented and recovery hastened in depression.[8] The practical problems of collecting a sufficient number of patients and the ethical problems of abstaining from treatment, both of which are necessary for randomized prospective studies, may prevent the necessary data from becoming available.

Current clinical experience clearly shows that the treatment of anxiety in suicidal patients is of utmost importance. A case history may illustrate this experience.

Case history

A 47-year-old divorced white man with bipolar disorder, which, before treatment, had cost him his career as an executive as a result of lapses in insight and judgement, had been stabilized on lithium and fluoxetine when he experienced a recurrence of depression, which occurred when he was under stress in a relationship and at the same time struggling to get a job in a new field. He noted the sudden onset of severe anxiety and feelings of dread and failure, became hopeless and attempted suicide by sitting in a closed garage in a car with the engine running. He was hospitalized and switched to venlafaxine 300 mg per 24 hours and alprazolam 4 mg per 24 hours. He had described every morning waking up to excruciating anxiety, which worsened when associated with hopelessness and fear of being unable ever to support himself and his children by his previous marriage. He noted the rapid onset of relief of his anxiety directly after the alprazolam doses in the morning, and over a few days his depression remitted. The patient has continued in remission on lithium 1500 mg, divalproex 1500 mg and venlafaxine 300 mg per 24 hours with the alprozolam tapered to an occasional 0.5 mg dose. He has successfully begun a new career.

References

1. Coryell W, Noyes R, Clancy J. Excess mortality in panic disorder. A comparison with primary unipolar depression. *Arch Gen Psychiatry* 1982;**39:**701–703.

2. Johnson J, Weissman MM, Klerman GL. Panic disorder, comorbidity and suicide attempts. *Arch Gen Psychiatry* 1990;**47:**805–808.

3. Angst J, Angst F, Stassen HH. Suicide risk in patients with major depressive disorder. *J Clin Psychiatry* 1999;**60(Suppl 2):**57–62.

4. Engstrom G, Persson B, Levander S. Temperament traits in male suicide attempts and violent offenders. *Eur Psychiatry* 1999;**14:** 278–283.

5. Fawcett J, Scheftner WA, Fogg L, et al. Time-related predictors of suicide in major affective disorder. *Am J Psychiatry* 1990;**147:** 1189–1194.

6. Fawcett J. Predictors of early suicide: identification and appropriate intervention. *J Clin Psychiatry* 1988;**49(Suppl 10):**7–8.

7. Henriksson MM, Isometsa ET, Kuoppasalmi KI, et al. Panic disorder in completed suicide. *J Clin Psychiatry* 1996;**57:** 275–281.

8. Fawcett J, Busch KA, Jacobs D, et al. Suicide: a four-pathway clinical–biochemical model. *Ann NY Acad Sci* 1997;**836:**288–301.

9. Busch KA, Clark DC, Fawcett J, Kravitz HM. Clinical features of inpatient suicide. *Psychiatr Ann* 1993;**23:**256–262.

10. Hall RC, Platt DE, Hall RC. Suicide risk assessment: a review of risk for suicide in 100 patients who made severe suicide attempts. Evaluation of suicide risk in a time of managed care. *Psychosomatics* 1999;**40:**18–27.

7
Eating disorders and suicide

Danuta Wasserman

Anorexia nervosa

Between 1 and 2% of teenage girls suffer from either anorexia nervosa (self-starvation) or bulimia (compulsive overeating), and these diagnoses are also being applied to a growing number of boys. Eating disorders have become more common in the past few decades. Anorexia often starts in conjunction with puberty; many children and adolescents go on slimming diets, and it is common for young people nowadays to be dissatisfied with their bodies and concerned with what they may and may not eat.[1,2,10] We live in a culture that promotes anorexic behaviour. Information intended to promote health by, for example, encouraging people to reduce their fat intake, cholesterol level and weight, has a negative impact on some susceptible people who lack the capacity for discrimination. They lose control over their own bodies and become inextricably caught up in their compulsive behaviour. Their images and perceptions of their own bodies are markedly disturbed and, in extreme cases, psychotic.[3,10]

Bulimia

Certain patients who are diagnosed as anorexic may alternate between anorexia and bulimic phases in which, without discernment and due to an inner compulsion, they consume all kinds of food and then promptly regurgitate it. Bulimics, like anorexics, cannot interpret signals from their body correctly, have difficulty in resisting obsessive impulses to starve themselves or grossly overeat, and lose control over their own body.[4]

Suicidality

Among people with eating disorders, crude mortality rates range between 6–8%, with suicide as the most common cause of death.[5,6] It is very common for young anorexics – girls and boys alike – to be depressed at the same time, and the risk of suicide is some 10 times higher (in some studies up to 20 times higher) among anorexic girls than among girls in general. Ethnic subcultures do not appear to exert any protective effect against anorexic behaviour.[7] Suicide risk remains high for many years after the initial assessment of eating disorders.[8,9] Very low weight at the time of the first assessment and frequent hospitalization are clear risk factors for suicide. Boys with eating disorders also run a markedly elevated risk of suicide and suicide attempts.

Comorbidity

People with eating disorders suffer often from depression. Substance and alcohol abuse with or without major depression are also common. This comorbidity increases the risk of suicide.[2,4] Girls and boys with eating disorders frequently have personality disorders. Anorexics with an obsessive–compulsive personality are introverted and often depressive. Aggressive retribution is a marked feature of their behaviour. This is the group in which the most severe cases of anorexia nervosa are encountered and in which the self-destructive acts take place. But anorexic patients with borderline and histrionic personalities may also run a risk of suicide despite their apparent openness and verbal skills. This is especially true when the patient is under the influence of alcohol or drugs, when impulse control is weakened.

Prevention and treatment

Beauty ideals that are conveyed in the media and often brought up by vacillating parents must be clarified by information and education at schools. It is natural to have some 'puppy fat' during puberty and for some years after puberty, owing to hormonal development. This natural process should not be counteracted by slimming. The parents should try to stop the slimming process or compulsive overeating in time before the severe compulsive behaviour develops.[10]

In the treatment of suicidal people with eating disorders, the usual methods of behavioural therapy combined with medication are advisable. These techniques should also be combined with some form of insight therapy, depending on the patient's intellectual ability, in order to clarify the psychodynamic aspects on both the personal and the relationship level.[4]

There are several conceivable psychological explanations for eating disorders. Starving oneself or overeating compulsively means making oneself the focus of attention and receiving care from others, while simultaneously rejecting this strongly. Eating disorders may be seen as a protest against relationships and as a means of controlling them, as well as an expression of a flight from reality and the erection of a barrier between oneself and the rest of the world. At a symbolic level, not eating or vomiting what one has already swallowed may also mean exerting control of one's intake and thereby meeting and controlling cultural pressure that urges the ideal of abstinence and labels self-indulgence as indicative of inadequacy and laziness. Paradoxically, with this behaviour, which is so much a matter of control, sufferers lose control of their bodies and feelings, and eventually lose their lives.

Another explanation – one that is outside the scope of relationships but that applies to the individual – may be that the growing girl wishes to curb her emerging womanliness, or the boy his manliness, as a protest against growing up. These young people may perhaps believe that mastering their oral needs to eat may also enable them to curb their sexual urges.

Teaching adolescents to appreciate themselves, to be contented with the way that they look and to be able to resist the ideals of slimness, which are out of all proportion in our culture, may be a protracted process.

Case history:
Not beautiful enough

Gunilla, aged 28

Gunilla had first attempted suicide by slitting her wrists at the age of 17 after her father's suicide. During her childhood, her father had repeatedly attempted suicide. Her mother had alcohol problems. The patient's sister, now a well-adjusted family therapist, had also tried to take her own life after failing on her first attempt to matriculate from upper secondary school.

Gunilla had lived with her paternal grandmother as a child, between the ages of 7 and 15. Her grandmother, who came from a farming family, had been anxious that Gunilla should eat properly and behave in an exemplary way. Gunilla had felt that her looks were all that mattered and that unless she was well dressed and her hair curled like a doll she was not loved. While living with her grandmother, she had fallen prey to minor eating disturbances. These increased in severity when she moved to live with her parents at the age of 15. She became pregnant at 18 and had an abortion. During that time, she found all food distasteful. She began suffering from anorexia, and successively developed bulimia as well.

Gunilla had always perceived herself as a failure – at school, in sports, as a friend and as a daughter. She had often changed schools because of her poor study results and she had never completed a course. Gunilla's elder siblings had all been to university. She felt that they had succeeded better in life than she had. Her relationship with her mother was the most fraught with conflict, and her relationships with her sisters were also troubled.

She had made her second suicide attempt at the age of 19, with several tranquillizers and sedatives. In a farewell letter addressed to her sister and mother, she had written that it would be better if she did not exist and wished her family happiness. She was reluctant to undergo any treatment after her suicide attempt.

Ten months later, owing to cardiac arrhythmia after an intense and protracted period of bulimia, she was once more admitted to hospital. Tests showed that she had impaired kidney function and that her arrhythmia was caused by disturbances in electrolyte balance. These somatic problems gave Gunilla a shock, and she now agreed to undergo psychological treatment.

Because she was diagnosed as suffering from severe depression, antidepressants were prescribed and she also embarked on psychotherapy. She thought she had been depressed for as long as she could remember, and she had become faddish about food long before puberty. Gunilla had always suffered from anxiety and been afraid to get too close to people. After 2 years' treatment, her abnormal eating habits were somewhat normalized. She still alternately went on slimming diets and indulged in overeating from time to time, but not as seriously as before.

At the age of 28, Gunilla married a man from Italy. She resumed her upper secondary school studies at evening courses but had no specific plans for the future.

References

1. Devaud C, Jeannin A, Narring F, et al. Eating disorders among female adolescents in Switzerland: prevalence and associations with mental and behavioral disorders. *Int J Eating Disord* 1998;**24**:207–216.

2. Fombonne E. Increased rates of psychosocial disorders in youth. *Eur Arch Psychiatry Clin Neurosci* 1998;**248**:14–21.

3. Favaro A, Santonastaso P. Purging behaviors, suicide attempts, and psychiatric symptoms in 398 eating disordered subjects. *Int J Eating Disord* 1996;**20**:99–103.

4. Schmidt U, Treasure J. The clinician's guide to getting better bit(e) by bit(e). London: Psychology Press; 1997.

5. Emborg C. Mortality and causes of death in eating disorders in Denmark 1970–1993: a case register study. *Int J Eating Disord* 1999;**25**:243–251.

6. Neumarker KJ. Mortality and sudden death in anorexia nervosa. *Int J Eating Disord* 1997;**21**:205–212.

7. French SA, Story M, Neumark-Sztainer D, et al. Ethnic differences in psychosocial and health

behavior correlates dieting, purging, and binge eating in population based sample of adolescent females. *Int J Eating Disord* 1997;**22:** 315–322.

8. Nielsen S, Moller-Madsen S, Isager T, et al. Standardized mortality in eating disorders: a quantitative summary of previously published and new evidence. *J Psychosom Res* 1998; **44:**413–434.

9. Patton GC. Mortality in eating disorders. *Psychol Med* 1988;**18:** 947–951.

10. Treasure J. Anorexia nervosa. A survival guide for families, friends and sufferers. London: Psychology Press; 1997.

8
Adjustment disorder and suicide

Danuta Wasserman

In the overwhelming majority of suicide cases a definite mental illness (e.g. depression, substance abuse of one kind or another, schizophrenia) may be found in the anamnesis. Nevertheless, a minority (some 10%) of people who commit suicide exhibit no open psychiatric symptoms or psychopathological features at the time of death. Apter et al.[1] showed that suicide may occur among young men 'in the absence of apparent psychopathology'. A Finnish study[2] found that young men with the diagnosis of adjustment disorder who committed suicide often communicated their suicidal thoughts to others, but that these thoughts were not taken seriously. These young men had a history of minor depressions of a short-lived nature, but no history of previous psychiatric treatment.

Suicide without recognizable psychopathology also occurs in elderly people who cannot cope with a major change in his or her life situation. A serious warning sign is an attempted suicide with a violent method in an elderly man or woman. If not appropriately managed, a suicide within a short time after such an attempted suicide often occurs.

Common symptoms of adjustment disorder are despondency, a sense of hopelessness, the feeling that one is not functioning as usual, and being close to tears. Anxiety is also common. These symptoms, which are natural as a reaction to severe grief or trauma, normally last no longer than 6 months and they usually cease when the person's life situation stabilizes and the stressor is eliminated. However, chronic states may occur, partly because the consequences of a trying life event or the trauma may persist. In a chronic traumatic situation of this kind, a new and stressful life event may be the last straw that precipitates the suicidal act.

Both young and elderly persons who commit suicide and have a diagnosis of adjustment disorder are usually fragile, sensitive, easily hurt and susceptible to stress.[3]

Since boys and men are often poor communicators, it is important to be observant of any signs of suicidal thoughts or depressive symptoms that are conveyed indirectly. The depressed youth refers not to his anxiety, sorrow or despondency, but to his failure to cope in ordinary situations – in family life, with friends, at school or work, in military service and in leisure activities, for example. It is advisable for depressive symptoms in boys and men to be treated without all criteria for the diagnosis of depression necessarily being met.

Longitudinal follow-up studies of patients with adjustment disorder who underwent crisis intervention show that they do not run a higher risk of developing depressive symptoms or dying from suicide than the overall population.[4]

Case history:
A rape

Marie, aged 24

Marie had undergone a radical change. From being a positive, ambitious extrovert she had been transformed, for the past 2 months, into a nervous, negative, 'lazy' person with no energy or lust for life.

She had fallen deeply in love with a college student, but had left him because he had turned out to be both manipulative and insincere. Shortly afterwards, she had met a man of her own age through a 'lonely hearts' advertisement. At the end of their first date, he had more or less raped her.

After the rape Marie had felt defiled, disappointed and filled with anxiety. She had an insistent sense of hopelessness and a marked fear that no man would ever want to live with her. She blamed herself, on the grounds that it had been her own fault for letting the man into her flat.

Marie tried to carry on studying, but all the energy that she had once had was gone. Thoughts about the rape kept going round and round in her head. She found it difficult to tell anyone about what had happened, and felt unclean and inferior. She began isolating herself and sought consolation in the Internet. Eventually, the computer took over all her waking hours.

When thoughts about taking her own life became persistent and frightening, she e-mailed a plea for help to an agency that provided professional advice about the body, mind and health, signing off as 'Young and desperate'. She told the psychologist who contacted her – first by e-mail and, in due course, in person – about her advanced suicide plans and all the details of how she planned to kill herself. All she lacked was the means of doing so.

After 3 months' supportive psychotherapy, during which she worked through her emotions connected with the rape and her attitude to the opposite sex, she felt better and resumed her studies.

References

1. Apter A, Bleich A, King RA, et al. Death without warning? A clinical postmortem study of suicide in 43 Israeli adolescent males. *Arch Gen Psychiatry* 1993;**50:**138–142.

2. Marttunen M, Aro H, Henriksson M, Lönnqvist J. Adolescent suicides with adjustment disorders or no psychiatric diagnosis. *Eur J Child Adolesc Psychiatry* 1994;**3:**101–110.

3. Runeson BS. Youth suicides unknown to psychiatric care providers. *Suicide Life Threat Behav* 1992;**22:**494–503.

4. Bronisch T. Adjustment reactions: a long-term prospective and retrospective follow-up of former patients in a crisis intervention ward. *Acta Psychiatr Scand* 1991;**84:**86–93.

9
Schizophrenia, other psychotic states and suicide

Alec Roy

Introduction

Bleuler described the suicidal drive as 'the most serious of schizophrenic symptoms'. It is generally considered that up to 10% of schizophrenics die by committing suicide. Most schizophrenics who commit suicide do so during the first few years of their illness. Thus, schizophrenic suicides tend to be relatively young, and about 75% are unmarried and male. However, suicide is not uncommon among schizophrenics who have been sick for a long time and suddenly have lost social support (usually from parents and especially mothers), owing to parental death. Up to 50% have made a previous suicide attempt. Depressive symptoms are closely associated with their suicide. Only a small percentage kill themselves because of hallucinated instructions or to escape persecutory delusions. Up to one-third of schizophrenic suicides occur during the first few weeks and months after discharge from a hospitalization; another one-third occur while the patient is in hospital. Adverse life events, such as ejection from the family, are often experienced in the few weeks before the suicide.

Premorbid functioning and insight

It has been noted that some schizophrenic suicide victims show high premorbid achievement, high self-expectations of performance and high awareness of their illness. It is thought that 'Given their inability to achieve major life goals, they felt inadequate, feared further deterioration of their mental abilities and decided to end their lives rather than continue living with chronic mental illness'. The authors concluded that such patients 'are likely to experience hopelessness defined as negative expectancies about the future and other psychological features of depression'.[1]

Positive and negative symptoms and schizophrenic suicide

A follow-up study found that schizophrenic patients dead from suicide had significantly lower negative symptom severity at index admission than patients without suicidal behaviors.[2] However, two positive symptoms – suspiciousness and delusions – were more severe among the suicides. The paranoid schizophrenic subtype was associated with an elevated risk of suicide (12%) and the deficit subtype was associated with a reduced risk (1.5%) of suicide. It may be that social and emotional withdrawal counter the emergence of suicidality in patients with schizophrenia and that the deficit syndrome defines a group at relatively low risk of suicide. Prominent suspiciousness in the absence of negative symptoms may define a relatively high-risk group. Another 2-year follow-up study similarly found that psychotic symptoms predicted later suicidal activity in schizophrenics whereas deficit symptoms did not.

Depression and other risk factors for suicide in schizophrenia

Risk factors for suicide in schizophrenia include:[3–7]

- being young and male;
- having a relapsing illness;
- having been depressed in the past;
- being currently depressed;
- having been recently admitted to hospital with accompanying depressive symptoms or suicidal ideas;
- having recently changed from in-patient to out-patient care; and
- being socially isolated in the community.

A US group set out to determine which of these risk factors distinguished schizophrenic suicides from living schizophrenic patients.[1] At their last hospitalization, significantly more of the eventual suicides were depressed (80%), felt inadequate (80%), felt hopeless (60%) and had suicidal ideation (73%). They found that being young, male and having a chronic illness with numerous exacerbations and remissions (a mean 6.8 admissions during a mean 8.4 years of illness) are the factors that distinguish schizophrenic suicides from living schizophrenic patients.

Prediction of suicide in schizophrenia

A recent study from the Phipps Clinic in Baltimore reported a mean 11-year follow-up on 1212 schizophrenics who were hospitalized between 1913 and 1940.[8] Twenty-eight of these 1212 patients (2%) committed suicide. When they were compared with those who did not suicide, they differed significantly in that they had more:

- previous suicide attempts;
- depression while hospitalized;
- suicidal thoughts during hospitalization;
- close relatives with affective illness;
- poor premorbid work and social histories;
- sexual worries; and
- psychomotor agitation during hospitalization.

Relationship of suicide to antipsychotic treatment

As part of the Finnish National Suicide Prevention Project all suicide victims with schizophrenia diagnosed according to the Diagnostic and Statistical Manual of Mental Disorders (DSM)-III-R who had a known treatment contact were classified according to the phase of illness (active or residual) and treatment (in-patient, recent discharge or other).[9] Characteristics of victims in terms of known risk factors for suicide in schizophrenia, as well as adequacy of neuroleptic treatment, were examined. It was found that 57% had active-phase schizophrenia and were not prescribed adequate neuroleptic treatment or were non-compliant, and 23% were estimated to be compliant non-responders. In-patient suicide victims had the highest proportion of negative or indifferent treatment attitudes (81%), whereas recently discharged suicide victims had the highest prevalence of comorbid alcoholism (36%), paranoid subtype (57%), recent suicidal behaviour or communication (74%), as well as the highest number of hospitalizations per year during their illness course and the shortest last hospitalization.

The Finnish study concluded that suicide risk factors may vary in different treatment phases of schizophrenia. Thus, substantial numbers of schizophrenic suicide victims are not receiving adequate neuroleptic medication, are non-compliant or do not respond to adequate doses of typical antipsychotic medication. Adequacy of antipsychotic treatment, particularly in the active phase, may be an important factor in suicide prevention among patients with schizophrenia.

Prevention of suicide in schizophrenia

Treatment of schizophrenia

Recently, it was reported that clozapine, an atypical neuroleptic, reduced suicidal behaviour in patients with schizophrenia.[10] Eighty-eight schizophrenic patients who were resistant to treatment with typical neuroleptics were treated with clozapine and prospectively evaluated for suicidality for periods of 6 months to 7 years. Clozapine treatment during the follow-up period resulted in markedly less suicidality. The number of suicide attempts with a high probability of success decreased from five to zero. The decrease in suicidality was also associated with improvement in depression and hopelessness. In another study comparing two atypical neuroleptics it was found that the rate of suicide attempts was significantly lower with olanzapine than with risperidone (0.6% versus 4.2%, $p = 0.029$).

However, the currently available data are not strong enough to allow firm recommendations about the use of atypical neuroleptics in suicidal schizophrenics.

Treatment of comorbidity

The majority of schizophrenic patients who commit suicide have depressive symptoms.[3-6] Studies have shown that both tricyclic antidepressants and selective serotonin reuptake inhibitors treat depressive symptoms in schizophrenia. It has recently been reported that treatment with olanzapine, an atypical neuroleptic, led to a significantly greater reduction in depressive symptoms in schizophrenics than treatment with haloperidol.

Another important comorbidity in suicidal schizophrenics is substance abuse, which requires vigorous treatment in schizophrenics who are at increased risk of suicidal behaviour.[11]

Psychosocial rehabilitation programmes

Intensive and tailor made social rehabilitation programmes are especially important for schizophrenic patients who often are very lonely and easily marginalized, either because of a lack of relatives or because relatives and friends are not always emotionally well prepared to be engaged in the schizophrenic's life.

Other psychotic states

Patients with schizoaffective disorder and other psychotic disorders are also at raised risk of suicide.[12,13] Their risk factors for suicide are similar to those described for the schizophrenic patient and include particularly having made a previous suicide attempt, being male, suffering from episodes of major depression and having substance abuse comorbidity. The postdischarge period is a period of increased risk, and non-compliance with treatment and inadequate treatment are also important risk factors.

Case report

MH was a 26-year-old single, unemployed man. He had his first psychiatric admission at the age of 19 when he began to hear voices and developed paranoid delusions. At that first admission he was also found to be depressed and had marked suicidal ideas. In the subsequent 7 years he had six psychiatric admissions – usually through the emergency room because of suicidal ideation or attempts and depression that accompanied exacerbations of the voices and delusions, which occurred when he was non-compliant with his neuroleptic medication. In between admissions he had been unable to find employment and had alienated his family.

In his last year of life he was living in a boarding house and was socially isolated. His last admission was precipitated when he tried to set fire to himself in his room in the boarding house. At admission he was very depressed, hopeless and paranoid. During the admission his psychotic symptoms attenuated when neuroleptic medication was reinstated. At discharge he was still somewhat depressed and he failed to attend his first follow-up out-patient appointment. A telephone call to the boarding house revealed that he had hanged himself in his room 2 days before the appointment.

References

1. Drake R, Gates C, Cotton P. Suicide among schizophrenics: a comparision of attempters and completed suicides. *Brit J Psychiatry* 1986;**149:**784–787.

2. Westermeyer J, Harrow M, Marengo J. Risk for suicide in schizophrenia and other psychotic and nonpsychotic disorders. *J Nerv Ment Dis* 1991; **179:**259–266.

3. Roy A (ed). Suicide. Baltimore: Williams and Wilkins; 1986.

4. Addington D, Addington J. Attempted suicide and depression in schizophrenia. *Acta Psychiatr Scand* 1992;**85:**288–291.

5. Dassori A, Mezzich J, Keshavan M. Suicidal indicators in schizophrenia. *Acta Psychiatr Scand* 1990;**81:**409–413.

6. Heila H, Isometsa E, Henriksson M, Heikkinen M, Marttunen M, Lönnqvist J. Suicide and schizophrenia: a nationwide psychological autopsy study on age- and sex-specific clinical characteristics of 92 suicide victims with schizophrenia. *Am J Psychiatry* 1997;**154:**1235–1242.

7. Rossau C, Mortensen P. Risk factors for suicide in patients with schizophrenia: nested case-control study. *Br J Psychiatry* 1997;**171:**355–359.

8. Stephens J, Richard P, McHugh P. Suicide in patients hospitalized for schizophrenia: 1913–1940. *J Nerv Ment Dis* 1999;**187:**10–14.

9. Heila H, Isometsa E, Henriksson M, et al Suicide victims with schizophrenia in different treatment phases and adequacy of antipsychotic medication. *J Clin Psychiatry* 1999;**60:**200–208.

10. Meltzer H, Okayli G. Reduction of suicidality during clozapine treatment of neuroleptic-resistant schizophrenics: impact on risk-benefit assessment. *Am J Psychiatry* 1995;**152:**183–190.

11. Verdoux V, Liraud F, Gonzales B, et al. Suicidality and substance misuse in first admitted subjects with psychotic disorders. *Acta Psychiatr Scand* 1999;**100:**389–395.

12. Radomsky E, Haas G, Mann JJ, Sweeney J. Suicidal behavior in patients with schizophrenia and other psychotic disorders. *Am J Psychiatry* 1999;**156:**1590–1595.

13. Stefenson A, Cullberg J. Committed suicide in a total schizophrenic cohort: in search of the suicidal process. *Nordic J Psychiatry* 1995;**49:**429–437.

IIIB
Personality disorders

10
Personality disorders and suicide

Danuta Wasserman

Introduction

The findings of psychological autopsy studies show that 'personality disorder' as the principal diagnosis is reported in approximately 9% of people who take their own lives, and 'abnormal personality' in up to 30%. However, figures as high as 34% for 'principal diagnosis of personality disorder' and up to 70% for 'abnormal personality' are also cited.[1]

The diagnosis of 'personality disorder' poses several methodological problems, and the incidence of personality disorders found among people who commit suicide varies depending on which patients are surveyed and the survey methods used. A restrictive approach is recommended, especially with the borderline diagnosis, more particularly in adolescents.[2] Every sign of borderline disorder may be manifested in connection with pubertal crises. Pregnant women or people in extreme life situations may also show clear borderline traits that later disappear.

Some personality disorders of particular importance in the therapeutic process, in terms of suicide prevention, are described below. Multiple personality disorders are not unusual, especially among young and middle-aged suicide victims.

Borderline personality

According to some cohort surveys of patients with the diagnosis of borderline personality disorder, up to 9% die from suicide.[3] Borderline personality is characterized by marked identity disturbance, with a chronic subjective sense of emptiness and difficulties in achieving steady, close relationships with others. Self-perceptions are full of contradictions, with repercussions on self-image, sexual orientation, long-term goals and choice of friends and occupation.

The mechanism known as 'splitting', the purpose of which is to keep bad and good impulses apart, is used as an essential psychological defence by persons with borderline personality. Since borderline personalities have difficulty in distinguishing between their own and others' good and bad impulses and emotions they may use 'projective identifications' (i.e. ascribe to others their own rage or the feeling that they wish to get rid of).

Patterns of unstable swings between extremes, with disparagement and overestimation, emotional lability, inadequate control of aggressive impulses, irascibility, and intense efforts to avoid separations – real and imagined – characterize people with borderline personality disorder. Their suicides often take place in a mood of fury mingled with despair triggered by separation from partners or significant others or because of an alteration in their accustomed lifestyle.[4,5]

Antisocial personality

The antisocial (or 'dis-social') person resembles the person with borderline personality disorder in many respects.[4–6] The specific additional traits of the antisocial personality are defective development of moral and ethical values, with a lack of empathy, an egocentric focus on one's own perceptual world and contempt for others.

People with an antisocial personality uninhibitedly act out their drives, impulses and aggressive fantasies. This behaviour is highly resistant to modification. Their dissatisfaction is transformed into aggressive action, sometimes directed against others and sometimes self-directed, rather than into signal anxiety, which has a normative and inhibiting role.

Suicide takes place in the rage that these people feel when, for example, they are apprehended for offences, embezzlement or crimes.

Narcissistic personality

The term 'narcissistic' is derived from the Greek myth of Narkissos, who was unable to stop contemplating his reflection in the waters of a spring. He had fallen so much in love with it that he eventually pined away and died.

Characteristic of this personality type is a paradoxical splitting between two entirely opposed self-images – one grandiose, making life a constant quest for confirmation of one's greatness with consequent effort to prove this, the other the antithesis of this, with a self-image full of shame, hate and terror of self-rejection. The experiential and conceptual world of narcissistic people are divided into the idyllic and the terrifying, which may alternate. Those in the surrounding world may also be perceived as representatives of one or the other sphere and so be idealized or disparaged. Ideas or people are rejected when they no longer provide a boost to the narcissistic person's self-image. The narcissistic personality also resembles both the borderline and the antisocial personality, with the major difference being that narcissistic people, when provoked, explode in outbursts of rage or aggressive behaviour only when the social situation permits.

Suicide may be the narcissist's reaction to losing his or her grandiose image (e.g. when ageing or illness destroys youthful charm or attractiveness, when a fall in social status or financial loss is incurred or when a well-regarded job or partner that imparted the reality or illusion of greatness is lost).[7,8]

Histrionic personality

The histrionic personality shows a consistent pattern of exaggerated emotionality and an endeavour to gain attention. A poor ability to read other people's intentions and needs contributes to disappointments being felt much more acutely than the actual facts justify. Perseverance, adjustment and contentment may be easily subverted by setbacks. Strains and disappointments bring a depressive, hopeless and helpless frame of mind.

Histrionic people commit suicide as a result of profound disappointment when they perceive strongly that they are no longer needed (e.g. because of the death of a loved one, restructuring at the workplace, or emigration due to unemployment, lack of friends, etc.). For very lonely people, separation from a pet such as a beloved dog may provide the trigger,

Anancastic personality

People with anancastic personality are highly orderly, conscientious and responsible but, unfortunately, easily frustrated, vulnerable, depressive and lonely, owing to their reserved attitude and their endeavours to set themselves apart from their peers. Perfectionist and knowledgeable, they lack tolerance of people who are ignorant and ordinary. There is often a gap between their aspirations and accomplishments, and they suffer from emotional and also intellectual instability, with ups and downs in terms both of affect and intellectual performance.

Many such people feel dissatisfied with their lives and are characterized by a tendency towards counterproductive behaviour, especially leaving others in order to avoid others leaving them. This is reflected both in their relationships and at work. Rejecting others before they can be rejected themselves may be these people's guiding principle. Towards themselves, they are denying and non-permissive. Despite their loneliness, they yearn for company and to belong to a group; but this desire may be thwarted by their need to dominate and exert control over others.

Suicidal acts take place when these people are experiencing deep downs and the prospects of bouncing back are perceived to be, or genuinely are, slim.

Other personality traits

The personality disorders described above, together with the emotionally unstable and anxious types of personality,[9] are the most prevalent among people who commit suicide. However, personality traits or disorders of paranoid, schizoid and obsessive–compulsive types are also found among suicide victims.

Childhood moulding

Many people with the personality types described above who take their own lives have had a childhood in which may be traced deficient parental care, often with a negative emotional climate and neglect of their most profound needs of closeness, contact, warmth and understanding. Alternatively, they may have been pathologically restrained, with their need to grow and develop through questioning and the ordinary frustrations of life thwarted during their upbringing.

Inadequate parental care may be due to the parents' inability to perceive the child's needs, the parents' moodiness or strictness or the child's lack of a close relationship when the parents die prematurely and there is no one to take their place as a secure substitute and good identification object or role model.

Severely distorted male or female identity, weak self-esteem and the superego, with elements of strong hostility to the self-image, is the result. Hostility (with risk of suicide) makes itself strongly felt in situations in which the person's low self-esteem is mercilessly exposed.

Genetic make-up

In families in which suicides take place, there are traditions of resolving conflicts or difficult situations by means of suicidal acts. Models like this pave the way for the child to adopt the same self-destructive strategies later in life. But hereditary factors also have a great bearing. Although the extent to which genetic components are implicated in suicide is debatable, there is much evidence pointing to their existence (see Chapter 3). Studies of my group show that people with low stress tolerance and high levels of anger and hostility have polymorphism on the tyrosine hydroxylase gene.[10] Tyrosine hydroxylase is an enzyme that governs the synthesis of noradrenaline (norepinephrine) and dopamine. Noradrenaline is a neurotransmitter that plays a part in the analysis of information received by the brain from various sensory organs. Accordingly, disturbances in the noradrenergic system may explain some cognitive disturbances. One hypothesis is that the polymorphism of the tyrosine hydroxylase gene may account for a basically low rate of activity in the noradrenergic system or for excessively low noradrenaline metabolism, and that this has consequences in stress-induced situations that call for increased attentiveness. When negative life events pile up, cognition deteriorates and, instead of finding an appropriate strategy, the person reacts, with anxiety, panic and rigidity. Typically, people on the brink of suicide have tunnel vision, are unable to make subtle distinctions, find solutions and be flexible, and perceive only the dark side of life (see Chapter 14).

Clinical manifestations of genetic predisposition depend on age[11] and on environmental factors, which vary from one phase of the human life cycle to another. This is why negative life events exert influence not only in childhood, but throughout a person's life. In the elderly, these events may coincide with other maturation-associated biochemical changes and altered brain functioning.

Suicide risk

People with personality disorders who take their own lives have, to a significantly greater extent than others, experienced a range of highly adverse life events such as troubles at work, unemployment, financial problems, family discord, lack of a permanent home, court convictions and separations. Problems often come to a head in the last week before the suicide, which precipitates the act (see Chapter 13).

The suicidal situation is often triggered by a primitive anger or a sense of hopelessness, or a blend of the two, when self-esteem is under severe threat and the usual self-image is unsustainable. When people's images of themselves and their existence collapses and cannot be reinstated in a normal grief process, there is a major risk of suicide. This applies particularly if there have been examples and models of suicidal behaviour in the family. However, suicidal impulses may subside and suicide risk diminish if new circumstances and therapeutic help appear and serve the purpose of providing the support and security that suicidal people are, for the time being, unable to generate for themselves.

Comorbidity

When one or more personality disorders and a psychiatric illness are present at the same time, the suicide risk is high.[6,12] Depression may sometimes be hard to detect in suicidal people with personality disorders since their feelings of hopelessness are relatively well concealed, even if their depression and despair are profound.

Treatment

Pharmacological treatment

Medication can be helpful in mitigating emotional instability, insecurity, easily aroused emotions, anxiety and rage.[13] Controlled studies show that low-dose antipsychotic drugs bring an improvement in a broad spectrum of different symptoms of severe borderline personality disorder and schizotypal personality disorder. Those who show aggressive behaviour respond to lithium. Patients with borderline and histrionic personality disorders who have suicidal tendencies respond to maintenance doses of antipsychotic drugs.

Carbamazepine has proved efficacious in reducing episodes of dyscontrol in patients with behavioural disturbances and borderline personality. Certain preparations (such as alprazolam) may cause loss of control and exacerbate suicidality in people with a borderline personality structure (see also Chapter 20).

Psychotherapy

Lasting and severe traumas during childhood affect personality development and have repercussions on experiences and the regulation of emotions. However, it is possible by different psychotherapeutic methods, both cognitive-behavioural[14] and psychodynamic,[15] to remedy a constantly recurring feeling of insecurity and unfulfilled emotional needs that are repeatedly brought to the fore in new stressful and traumatic situations that arise later in life.

During treatment, it is important to work through the old and new traumas and show how the current emotional reactions are a repetition of previous emotional reactions. In this kind of treatment, the cultural factors that influence people's behaviour and emotional expressions must also be taken into account. Efforts to motivate the patient to receive drug treatment, when necessary, should also be included in psychotherapeutic treatment (see also Chapter 19).

Prevention

Research shows that, for patients with personality disorders, the prognosis is good with respect to both the psychiatric illness itself and their suicidality if, during the turbulent years of their youth and early adulthood, they succeed in improving their affect and impulse management. For patients with such characteristics as warmth, charm, attractiveness, talent and high intelligence, the prognosis is better than for others.[16]

Chronic suicidality, with repeated suicide attempts, does not necessarily mean that the patient will die from suicide. Active and prompt intervention, with both pharmacological and psychotherapeutic treatment, in response to acute problems such as interpersonal or work difficulties, can save the lives of vulnerable and suicidal people. Those who have attempted suicide previously should be taught to seek psychiatric help in time.

References

1. Isometsä ET, Henriksson MM, Heikkinen ME, et al. Suicide among subjects with personality disorders. *Am J Psychiatry* 1996;**153:**667–673.

2. Brent DA, Johnson BA, Perper J, et al. Personality disorder, personality traits, impulsive violence and completed suicide in adolescents. *J Am Acad Child Adolesc Psychiatry* 1994;**33:**1080–1086.

3. Modestin J. Completed suicide in personality disordered inpatients. *J Pers Disord* 1989;**3:**113–121.

4. Kjelsberg E, Eikeseth PH, Dahl AA. Suicide in borderline patients: predictive factors. *Acta Psychiatr Scand* 1991;**84:**283–287.

5. Kullgren G. Factors associated with completed suicide in borderline personality disorder. *J Nerv Ment Dis* 1988;**176:**40–44.

6. Kjellander C, Bongar B, King A. Suicidality in borderline personality disorder. *Crisis* 1998;**19:** 125–135.

7. Clark DC. Narcissistic crises of aging and suicidal despair. *Suicide Life Threat Behav* 1993; **23:**21–26.

8. Ronningstam EF, Maltsberger JT. Pathological narcissism and sudden suicide-related collapse. *Suicide Life Threat Behav* 1998; **28:**261–271.

9. Cheng AT, Mann AH, Chan KA. Personality disorder and suicide. A case-control study. *Br J Psychiatry* 1997;**170:**441–446.

10. Persson ML, Wasserman D, Geijer T, et al. Tyrosine hydroxylase allelic distribution in suicide attempters. *Psychiatry Res* 1997;**72:**73–80.

11. Duberstein PR, Conwell Y, Caine ED. Age differences in the personality characteristics of suicide completers: preliminary findings from a psychological autopsy study. *Psychiatry* 1994;**57:** 213–224.

12. Angst J, Clayton PJ. Personality, smoking and suicide: a prospective study. *J Affect Disord* 1998;**51:**55–62.

13. Hori A. Pharmacotherapy for personality disorders. *Psychiatry Clin Neurosci* 1998;**52:**13–19.

14. Linehan M, Armstrong H, Suarez A, et al. Cognitive–behavioral treatment of chronically parasuicidal

borderline patients. *Arch Gen Psychiatry* 1991;**48:**1060–1064.

15. Bateman A, Fonagy P. Effectiveness of partial hospitalization in the treatment of borderline personality disorder: a randomized controlled trial. *Am J Psychiatry* 1999;**156:**1563–1569.

16. Rothenhausler HB, Kapfhammer HP. Outcome in borderline disorders. A literature review. *Fortschritte der Neurologie-Psychiatrie* 1999;**67:**200–217.

IIIC
Somatic disorders

11
Physical illness and suicide

Jouko Lönnqvist

Health-care staff taken by surprise

The role of physical illness in suicide has received little attention in research and education. Although suicide is a rare event, elevated suicide risk is a known feature of many somatic disorders.[1] Most suicide victims consult health professionals for reasons of physical ill-health in the last 6 months of their lives. However, many of them do not express their suicidal ideation, or even their depressive feelings, in clear verbal terms.

Retrospective analysis after a suicide may afford knowledge of the suicidal person's many problems, but in many cases the act of suicide remains enigmatic. Suicide almost always arouses a mixture of feelings among health-care staff – anxiety, a sense of helplessness, anger, rage, sorrow, guilt and many other feelings. Numerous simple explanations may be offered. Suicide reminds health-care professionals of the limits of their care: the best possible help was not available and normal clinical practice was insufficient to prevent suicide. But could the unpredictable have been predicted? Does the suicide carry a message that we can learn for the future?

It is a challenge to improve both understanding of suicide risk and treatment of suicidal patients in clinical practice.

Physical illness and suicide risk

Epidemiological studies have revealed that a number of somatic illnesses are associated with elevated suicide risk.[1,2] The physical illnesses most commonly connected with suicide are:

- cancer;
- human immunodeficiency virus (HIV) infection and AIDS;
- stroke;
- juvenile diabetes mellitus;
- delirium;

- epilepsy;
- Parkinson's disease;
- traumatic brain damage;
- spinal cord injury;
- multiple sclerosis;
- Huntington's disease; and
- amyotrophic lateral sclerosis.

Chronic states, disability and negative prognosis are correlated with suicide. Certain somatic markers, such as low serum cholesterol, also appear to be associated with high suicide risk.[3]

In addition, some people who eventually commit suicide suffer not only from severe depression but also from an intense fear of severe somatic illness, such as cancer or HIV infection. This kind of hypochondria usually leads to numerous health-care consultations, with physical examinations yielding negative results and, in turn, bringing disappointment and a growing sense of hopelessness and helplessness. The many faces of depression, especially when psychosomatic symptoms are present, can mislead even experienced clinicians and cause misunderstandings between patients and their doctors.

Mental retardation and dementia, on the other hand, are two severe organic brain disorders associated with a reduced risk of suicide.[4]

Physical illness and the suicidal process

The events that culminate in suicide, which involve suicidal ideation and often attempted suicide as well, are known as the 'suicidal process' (see Chapter 2). Suicide is the fatal outcome of what is, as a rule, a long-term process shaped by various interacting genetic, biological, physiological, cognitive, emotional, behavioural, situational, social, societal and cultural factors. In this process, physical illness may be seen as either a long-term risk factor or a more immediate, precipitating cause.

In the first 5 years of cancer, for example, the probability of suicide is elevated. Suicide risk is clearly highest in the first few months after diagnosis, when the adaptation crisis has not yet been resolved. In many other chronic and progressive somatic diseases, the risk may fluctuate depending on the course of the illness. Exacerbation or deterioration of a somatic disease may often also trigger a suicidal crisis. However, most people are capable of living and working through even the most threatening stages of illness if support is available from their significant others and the health-care system. Despite the tremendous acute stress and chronic adaptational demands associated with all major somatic disorders, surprisingly few sufferers from severe physical illness actually commit suicide.

In terms of social background, family status and previous suicidality, as well as psychiatric diagnoses and personality characteristics, patients with somatic disease who commit suicide are usually clinically very similar to other suicide victims, their main problems being depressive mood and adaptational difficulties. Suicide risk is indirectly associated with physical illness through the anxiety, depression, narcissistic rage, pain, fear and side effects of treatment, substance or alcohol abuse or delirious states experienced by the sick person. Loneliness and isolation that ensue from the illness, access to lethal suicide methods, and imitation of other suicides are other important factors in this context. Elevated suicide risk is not normally directly related to the somatic illness but, rather, is due to associated comorbidity. If this comorbidity remains undetected, the patient's distorted behaviour may further accelerate the suicide process.

The best predictive risk factors for suicide among patients suffering from physical illnesses are previous suicide attempts, anorexia nervosa, depression, psychosis, substance abuse and personality disorder. However, the high suicide risk associated with physical illness is mediated through many mechanisms.

First, since terminal illness makes death an imminent reality, it may prompt patients with incurable diseases to avoid or even flee from the feared end of their lives, with the prospect of pain, anxiety and annihilation. Some prefer to choose their mode of death actively, by suicide. Proponents of assisted suicide make use in their arguments of these strong emotional reactions that arise in people who know they are dying. However, the idea of assisted suicide is undoubtedly dangerous given that adequate somatic and psychiatric treatment has seldom been available to terminally ill suicide victims.

Secondly, the idea of increasing dependence on others as a result of illness may be the force that drives some patients to commit suicide.

Thirdly, a physical illness often implies the threat of a future in which the health-care system, rather than relatives, will take care of the patient. Separation from loved ones may be a patient's dominant fear. Suicidal ideation that is expressed and openly received by significant others is the most obvious factor prompting early intervention.

Physical illness and somatopsychiatric comorbidity in completed suicide

The 'psychological autopsy' is a comprehensive method of investigating the background to a completed suicide by studying all available data and the role of the physical illness in the suicide. The prevalence of physical disorders found in psychological autopsy studies has varied widely between 16 and 70%. A recent Scottish case-control study identified physical ill-health as one of the major factors that is independently associated with suicide, and treatment of mental disorders comorbid with physical ill-health was seen as an important strategy in suicide prevention.[5] In a nationwide Finnish psychological autopsy study, when the diagnosis of all potentially relevant physical disorders had been included, the incidence of somatic illness was found to be 46%, its most prevalent form being vascular disease.[6] A Finnish study of elderly suicide victims found that 88% had been suffering from physical illnesses.[7] These findings clearly indicate that somatopsychiatric comorbidity poses a special challenge for preventing suicide to doctors who treat elderly patients.

Four per cent of all suicide victims in a Finnish study were diagnosed as suffering from cancer, but only a small minority were terminally ill. The proportion of cancer patients who committed suicide and who had comorbid depressive syndromes was the same as that of the control suicide victims (four out of five), and the former very often had suicidal tendencies even before their cancer diagnosis. Only a very small minority of suicide victims suffering from cancer presented no comorbid mental disorder. These findings refute the idea that assisted suicide might serve as an appropriate means of helping severely ill somatic patients. As noted above, such an idea is undoubtedly dangerous, given that adequate somatic and psychiatric treatment is seldom, if ever, available.[8,9]

Suicide prevention through treatment of somatic diseases

Since physical illness is usually a concomitant or precipitating factor in the suicidal process, medical treatment of somatic illness is an important means of suicide prevention. Even a minor positive event may be life-saving when a patient stands on the brink of suicide. Good clinical practice invariably also means effective suicide prevention.

In clinical practice a doctor treats an individual patient, not just a specific illness. A somatically ill patient very often has other comorbid and mental problems, usually anxiety or depression, or both. Accordingly, only a tailor-made treatment strategy – a balanced, optimal treatment plan comprising somatic, psychological and social elements – can be effective. It is known that suicide victims never suffer from ordinary, simple problems. They tend to have several diagnoses, they are awkward and troublesome patients and they often have communication difficulties. They have problems in co-operating with health-care professionals and they question the ability of these professionals to help.

Most countries believe in a comprehensive suicide-prevention strategy (i.e. that all available means must be used to achieve an overall impact on suicide rates at the population level). Accordingly, all clinical specialists should be familiar with the high-risk groups in their own fields and the high-risk situations associated with specific somatic illnesses. This means, for example, that neurologists who treat patients with multiple sclerosis must be aware that such patients run a suicide risk that is twice as high as normal, that this risk fluctuates according to the course of the illness and the patients' mood, and that beta-interferon treatment, for example, may modify the risk. Likewise, all other specialists and, indeed, all doctors have their own specific points to ponder and their own challenges to meet in suicide prevention.

With the growing success of various somatic treatments in recent years, suicide risk has also declined. The most recent example is HIV infection and AIDS. Suicide risk among people who are HIV-positive has fallen markedly as the outcome has improved. Additional scientific research resulting in effective treatment of various physical illnesses will probably further reduce suicide risk. Good medical treatment of underlying somatic disease undoubtedly improves the scope for successful suicide prevention.

Case history:
'When the bullet hits – suffering in silence'

A middle-aged man who had suffered from urethral stricture for some years was hospitalized for surgery. The stricture was the result of a gonorrhoeal infection that he had contracted before his marriage, more than 10 years earlier. The urogenital infection preyed on his mind and he became anxious and depressed.

Shortly after the operation and discharge from the hospital, the patient hanged himself. He had been unable to face the overwhelming threat that he perceived his physical illness to imply. He had received proper surgical treatment for his urethral stricture, but his depression and anxiety had never been recognized or treated – he had been left alone with his fears.

One wonders what the 'reason' for this suicide was, what the precipitating factors were and what kinds of risk factor were present. It emerged afterwards (unfortunately not before or during his stay in hospital) that the patient's brother had committed suicide shortly before the appearance of the urogenital symptoms in the patient. This event had plunged the patient into profound grief. As the urethral stricture had developed, he had begun using painkillers in abundance. It was only discovered after his death that he had been resorting to painkillers occasionally over the past 10 years following a severe bullet wound that had caused an open brain injury to the left fronto-temporal sensorimotor region, with resultant post-traumatic epilepsy. The patient had resumed his work but had been obliged to take antiepileptic medication.

Despite his head injury and restricted work capacity, he had succeeded in achieving a happy marriage at the age of over 40 years and supporting his family, including a small child. The psychological autopsy revealed several other traumatic events in the patient's life that had never been worked through in any kind of psychological treatment. His father had died when the patient was 20 years old and his mother had died in childbirth. As a young man, the patient had had an illegitimate son, whom he abandoned.

We are still ignorant of the 'reason' for his suicide, since his thoughts and feelings are unknown to us. Was he afraid of losing his happy marriage because of impotence? Did he fear being left alone – as he had been by his mother as a baby, by his father as a young man and finally, recently, by his brother? These losses and the psychological experience of losing contact with his first child may have aroused in him the fear that his wife might leave him.

No one knows. Nevertheless, the patient's suicide risk could have been recognized if the doctor treating his epilepsy had noted his misuse of painkillers and the signs of depression and anxiety that had developed in connection with the urogenital problems.

References

1. Harris EC, Barraclough BM. Suicide as an outcome for medical disorders. *Medicine* 1994;**73:** 281–296.

2. Stenager EN, Stenager E. Physical illness and suicidal behaviour. In: Hawton K, van Heeringen K (eds). Suicide and attempted suicide. Chichester: John Wiley & Sons Ltd; 2000;405–420.

3. Partonen T, Haukka J, Virtamo J, et al. Association of low serum total cholesterol with major depression and suicide. *Br J Psychiatry* 1999;**175:** 259–262.

4. Harris EC, Barraclough B. Suicide as an outcome for mental disorders: a meta-analysis. *Br J Psychiatry* 1997;**170:**205–228.

5. Cavanagh JTO, Owens DGC, Johnstone EC. Suicide and undetermined death in south-east Scotland. A case-control study using the psychological autopsy method. *Psychol Med* 1999;**29:** 1141–1149.

6. Henriksson MM, Aro HM, Marttunen MJ, et al. Mental disorders and comorbidity in suicide. *Am J Psychiatry* 1993;**150:**935–940.

7. Henriksson MM, Marttunen MJ, Isometsä ET, et al. Mental disorders in elderly suicides. *Int Psychogeriatr* 1995;**7:**275–286.

8. Henriksson MM, Isometsä ET, Hietanen PS, et al. Mental disorders in cancer suicides. *J Affect Disord* 1995;**36:** 11–20.

9. Hietanen P, Lönnqvist J. Cancer and suicide. *Ann Oncol* 1991; **2:**19–23.

IIID
Social conditions

12
Some social dimensions of suicide

Ilkka Henrik Mäkinen and Danuta Wasserman

Introduction

Even if suicide is the result of an individual decision, it neither originates nor is committed in a vacuum. Thus, while social scientists are working to determine the relations between the structure or dynamics of societies and the number of suicides committed in them, it may also be useful for the individual medical practitioner to pay attention to the social environment in which the patient lives and suffers.

We choose to call these factors social, rather than societal or sociological, because they are clearly recognizable at the individual level. This makes them at least partly dependent on individual decisions. For the sake of convenience, we may sometimes use expressions that implicate a straightforward causality between various social factors and individual suicides. However, such a direct causality should not be inferred (see below). From the doctor's point of view the distinction, even if it is a necessary one for the scientist, is less important. If a patient belongs to a group in which suicide, for one reason or another, is more common than in other groups, then it is cause for vigilance on the part of the care-giver.

It has been argued that there are three basic determinants of population health in modern societies: material wealth, social structure and lifestyles. All of these are intertwined. As sheer material wealth in itself does not seem to be of great importance in relation to suicide, the role of the social structure is discussed below. The structure should, however, be understood in the context of the way in which structural roles (e.g. being married, receiving disability benefits or having recently migrated) may imply a certain type of lifestyle.

Social categories are inherently dynamic. Although a static mode of description is easier to communicate, one should remember that the human contents of the categories (and sometimes the categories themselves) are constantly changing. Sometimes the person's move into a 'risk category' is the most dangerous moment from the suicidological point of view. Individual-based research shows that many of the stressful or traumatic 'life events' are of such social origin.

Many social theories of suicide regard large-scale changes in the social environment as being of major importance for changes in suicide mortality levels. An important element in Émile Durkheim's famous theory of suicide[1] (1992) was the disruptive effect of rapid modernization. In the 1990s, drastic increases in suicide mortality have taken place in the former Soviet Union. They have been connected to the 'transitionary' nature of post-communist society, although the exact causal question has not yet been resolved.

Social environment in general

The first dimension to be considered is the individual's social network. All previous research points unambiguously to the conclusion that the ties that attach the individual to his or her peers and to the larger society are of utmost importance in relation to his or her propensity to commit suicide. The number, duration, strength and quality of social relations are all inversely related to suicide risk. People with marital, kinship, occupational, friendship or other types of social ties are generally at lower risk of committing suicide than those who lack these ties, and people who commit suicide generally possess fewer social ties of any kind in comparison with other people.[2,3,4] (See also Chapter 13.)

As with other social factors, the causality question is not clear-cut. A person may commit suicide because he or she lacks social ties, or he or she may experience loneliness because of some third factor (such as mental illness), which ultimately causes isolation and thus influences suicidality in several ways simultaneously. However, there is evidence to suggest that isolation, both physical and psychological, has an effect of its own that is independent of other circumstances.

There are notions of men's suicidality being more influenced by social circumstances than women's. In times when there are sudden movements in suicide mortality figures, men's suicide rates seem both to rise and to fall more steeply than women's. This could be interpreted as men having a greater propensity to react suicidally to external change. However, there is probably no great difference between the sexes when the crisis touches on the personal sphere (see also Chapter 14).

The presence of other people may mean that social support is available, and even if this is not the case, it may still provide an invisible but nonetheless effective form of social control. Community-oriented life also often implies that one's everyday activities follow a certain routine, which in itself works protectively. Should the worst come to the worst, many suicides are prevented by the purposeful or coincidental intervention of others. Furthermore, the preventive effect of social ties seems to be cumulative: divorced or widowed people have higher suicide rates than married people but among the divorced and widowed those who are not in a position to work or are unemployed, the suicide rates are even higher still.

However, the coin also has a reverse side. Social environments in which self-destructive behaviour seems to be valued (e.g. some hard-rock milieus) or in which many such acts are committed and reported may prove to be more detrimental to the individual than protective. Areas in which there are many suicide attempts are often also those in which various social problems accumulate. Living in a group and following its norms and behaviours is in many ways easier than trying to exist alone, but so too, in this respect, is dying.

Family relationships

Perhaps the most important social environment is the family. While its size may be diminishing and its authority, and even its legitimacy, are under attack in modern society, it still provides the individual with basic emotional security (or a lack of it) as well as social, and sometimes also financial, support. Furthermore, it still acts as a major institution in people's socialization and in the transmission of values and attitudes to the next generation.

There are clear and nearly universal differences in suicidality between people in different marital status groups. Married people generally have the lowest suicide rates, and divorced and widowed people have rates that are two or three times higher. The rate of suicide also seems to vary inversely with the duration of the marriage and the number of children in it. The suicide rates of unmarried people are also generally higher than those of married people.

Marital status (unlike, for example, age) is a voluntary category. Today it is not automatically assumed that a marriage should be lifelong. New categories, such as cohabitation without marriage, have appeared since the 1960s in many countries.

The difference between marital groups can even be observed at the collective level. Familistic areas, inhabited predominantly by married couples with children, generally have the lowest suicide rates in modern cities. Several factors are involved in the shaping of a familistic lifestyle. First, there is the selection into the married group, which tends to exclude the people who are most physically and psychologically vulnerable. Secondly, the fact of being married in modern society usually means that there is a degree of trust between the partners so that they choose to formalize their relationship instead of merely cohabiting. Thirdly, a family-centered life with children often takes place among other couples so that a social environment is created, which especially in the larger cities stands in stark contrast to the more irregular lifestyles in other areas. All these factors are likely to lower suicidality, partly through selection, and partly through protection. Therefore, a status change away from this category (e.g. through divorce) may involve a major risk for the individual.

However, being in a family does not automatically mean that a person is protected. As in other social environments, the functionality of the family is essential to its influence on individual suicidality. For example, people with a history of suicide in their families run a considerable surplus risk of committing the act themselves. However, not only the family, but even friends and acquaintances can exercise influence on individual suicidality.

Last but not least, marriage is also a cultural category. While Western marriages are supposedly based on romantic love, this is not an issue, or not at least the main determinant, in many other cultural environments. The opinions of parents and relatives, as well as economic factors, may greatly influence marriage decisions. This implies that the effect of marriage might not be exactly the same across different cultural groups. For example, the high suicide mortality among young females in the rural areas of China has been linked to the arranged marriages that they undergo and to the low status of the bride in her new family. In the past, there have also been societies in which the suicide of the survivors of 'great men' was the social norm. Although these practices are on the wane, the behaviour itself continues even in some contemporary relationships.

Employment

Another main sphere of life is that of one's occupation. There are disparities in suicidality between different categories, with the most important of them being those between those who are employed and those who are not employed. Research suggests that those who are not employed are a high-risk group for both suicide and suicide attempt;[5,6] however, the causality question has not been fully resolved.

As with a marriage, a job can provide many things. After the initial selection process, it may offer not only money but also social contacts, social position, support possibilities and stable routines. Understandably, the connection between unemployment and suicide is largely dependent on what exactly unemployment means for the individual. In the crisis years of the 1930s, unemployment peaks in the USA and in Western Europe would sometimes be visibly followed by peaks in (male) suicide rates, but in modern times, corresponding phenomena cannot be discerned at an aggregate level in the existing studies. This change can probably be explained by the development of financial support systems, which soften the consequences of unemployment. However, being a member of the group that remains unemployed regardless of economic trends may be indicative of grave personal or social problems.

When one person in an interdependent social unit, such as a family, becomes unemployed or otherwise leaves the labour market, it seldom affects him or her alone. Depending on economic or other circumstances, the effect on the whole family may vary from slight annoyance (or even relief) through to a major life crisis, which may eventually lead to suicidal behaviour.

Generally, people who are gainfully employed full-time seem to have the lowest suicide rates. The suicide risk of those who are not employed also depends on other factors: e.g. it is difficult to say to what extent the generally higher suicide rates among old people in most European countries can be explained by their retirement from working life alone. However, there are two special high-risk groups for suicide that can be easily recognized.

- people who are outside the labour market for other than home- or career-related reasons (e.g. those on a disabled pension); and
- the unemployed i.e. persons who would like to have a job but cannot find one.

Of these the first group seems to be at gravest risk.

There are also differences among the employed. Thus, although there may be variation between countries, most European research points at a 'class ladder' in suicide mortality. Among men, those holding higher 'white-collar' positions tend to have the lowest suicide rates; these rates increase with every successive step down the ladder and are highest on the bottom rung among 'unskilled' workers. The relationship is, of course, confounded by (and also due partly to) other socio-psychological and cultural differences between the holders of the status positions.

For women, the picture is not so clear-cut – there are indications of a U-shaped relationship, where those in the middle positions are at the lowest risk, while women in both the leading and lower positions demonstrate a higher level of suicidality. However, the classification of women's class positions in modern society is a subject of dispute among social scientists.

Moving and migration

It may be generally assumed that all changes in the social environment, to the extent that some important social ties are disrupted, are more or less suicide-promoting. Disregarding the question of causality, it seems that separations, divorces and negative changes in a person's labour status are connected with suicidal crises and ensuing actions. This is also true of geographical movement. A recent or repeated change of residence is often found to be more prevalent among people who kill themselves than among other people. Furthermore, areas that are characterized by high levels of mobility often have high suicide rates.

In relation to suicide and geographical movement, most research has focused on emigration–immigration (i.e. the move over international borders). Generally speaking, the suicide rates of immigrants tend to be higher in the new country than in the country of origin, a fact that can, in many cases, be accounted for by the 'negative selection' of the migrants (i.e. those with the least to lose move out) as well as by the general stress of immigration along with the psycho-social risks it entails.[7,8]

With regard to long-term developments, there is no coherent picture – there are reports of converging processes, whereby the suicide mortality of various immigrant groups moves gradually closer to that of the host population over time, but this does not appear to apply to all groups everywhere. For example, immigrant Finns in Sweden still experience a very high level of suicide mortality even after decades in their new country.

This last-mentioned fact illustrates the complexity of the issue. All over the world, people from numerous nations, all with their own migration (and suicide) traditions, emigrate for various reasons to the recipient states, which in turn receive them in different ways. In such circumstances, few general things can be said about the longer-term effects of such multiple processes on suicidality. However, it does appear as if the cultural background of the individual is of great importance. People from nations with low suicide rates (e.g. the Arabic and many Mediterranean and South American nations) tend to maintain the low suicide level in their new environment, while immigrants from Eastern Europe, for example, have a greater risk of suicide in their new countries.

No less important is the path of acculturation that the new immigrant chooses from the options available. A marginalized person, living on the outskirts of the host society, is very dependent on his closest social ties, whereas one striving for quick assimilation risks losing the support of his own group while perhaps not being readily accepted into the group to which he aspires to belong. Immigrants employing a common 'separation' strategy prefer to live among their own ethnic group after moving into the new society, which may very well be beneficial from the point of view of suicidality, as long as the group is large enough to provide support for them.

Culture and religion

Culture, in the sense of the collective ideas guiding the individual's behaviour, and perhaps its main constituent – religion, are social in the sense that they are most often absorbed in the society of one's origin. Having once been internalized, they often show a surprising ability to subsist in new environments through a process of creative adaptation. It seems that much of the difference in suicidal behaviour between national groups can be connected with differences in cultural outlook. Groups differ greatly in the cultural 'visibility' of suicide, the attitude that is taken towards it and the situations in which it may be considered as an acceptable course of action.[9-11] While this is not always visible at the individual level, it can be clearly seen at the collective level, where the rates of suicide, the distribution of suicide and the ways of and motives for committing the act, clearly separate different cultural spheres from each other.

An example of this can be found in the remarkable stability of suicide rates in different countries and areas. Even when suicide mortality in general increases or decreases, the *differences* between the units – their rank order, tend to remain more or less the same.[12] Although there are individual exceptions to this observation, a comparison of the current suicide rates of European nations to those of 100 years ago reveals surprisingly stable patterns, the origin of which must be sought in the differences amongst national and local cultures.

The young, however, constitute an exception of this rule, their suicide rates being more volatile than those of other age groups, perhaps owing to international influences.

Traditionally, religion has been considered to be the 'matrix' of culture. Its relation to suicidality became famous through Durkheim's study, in which he claimed that Roman Catholics always had lower suicide rates than Protestants. However, in modern societies religion has become individualized to such an extent that its effects can be better discerned between individuals than between societies. Personal religiosity is still the main determinant of *attitudes* towards suicide in Western Europe. In this respect, it seems to be strongly negatively connected with (non-) suicidal behaviour, as long as the religious attachment is balanced.[13]

Due to limitations of space, only the most important references have been added. For further information, the reader is well advised to consult the more general works in the area.[14-17]

References

1. Durkheim E. Suicide. London: Routledge; 1992.
2. Heikkinen ME, Isometsä ET, Marttunen MJ, et al. Social factors in suicide. *Br J Psychiatry* 1995;**167:**747–753.
3. Kreitman N. Suicide, age, and marital status. *Psychol Med* 1988; **18:**121–128.
4. Maris RW. Social and familial risk factors in suicidal behavior. *Psychiatr Clin North America. Review.* 1997;**20:**519–550.
5. Platt S. Suicidal behavior and unemployment. A literature review. Health policy implications of unem-

ployment. Geneva: World Health Organization; 1985: 87–132.

6. Norström T. The impact of alcohol, divorce, and unemployment on suicide: a multilevel analysis. *Soc Forces* 1995;74:293–314.

7. Whitlock FA. Migration and suicide. *Med J Aust* 1971;**2:** 840–848.

8. Johansson LM. Migration, mental health, and suicide. An epidemiological, psychiatric, and cross-cultural study. Stockholm: Department of Clinical Neuroscience and Family Medicine, Karolinska Institute; 1997.

9. Farberow NL (ed). Suicide in different cultures. Baltimore: University Park Press; 1975.

10. Mäkinen IH. Suicide-related crimes in contemporary European criminal laws. Crisis 1997;**18:** 35–47.

11. Kral MJ. Suicide as social logic. *Suicide Life Threat Behav* 1994; **24:**245–255.

12. Mäkinen IH, Wasserman D. Suicide prevention and cultural resistance: stability in European countries' suicide ranking, 1970–1988. *Ital J Suicidol* 1997; **7:**73–85.

13. Pescosolido B, Georgianna S. Durkheim, suicide, and religion: toward a network theory of suicide. *Am Soc Rev* 1989;**54:**33–48.

14. Dublin LI. Suicide. A sociological and statistical study. New York: Ronald Press; 1963

15. Lester D (ed). Le suicide: 100 years later. Philadelphia: Charles Press; 1994.

16. Mann JJ (ed). Suicide. The psychiatric clinics of North America, vol 20. Philadelphia: WB Saunders; 1997.

17. Pritchard C. Suicide: the ultimate rejection? A psycho-social study. Buckingham, UK: Open University Press; 1995.

Section IV
Risk situations for suicide and risk assessment

13

Negative life events (losses, changes, traumas and narcissistic injury) and suicide

Danuta Wasserman

Introduction

Fortunately, suicide is a rare occurrence. Although many people find themselves in the kinds of situation described below, only a small minority choose suicide. This chapter contains an account of various risk situations, any one of which may be 'the last straw' – the stressor that prompts a vulnerable person to commit a suicidal act. Feeling loved, a sense of belonging, being needed and respected by others and an awareness of one's own worth are important to all human beings. Negative life events prevent the satisfaction of these basic needs and may bring some people close to suicide. This applies to those who have no means of regaining what they have lost and who, at the same time, perceive indifference, rejection or aggression among the people around them.

In a suicidal person, life and death wishes vie for supremacy. The person's ambivalence in other respects may be just as marked. Current negative life events are often superimposed on the experience of similar events in childhood or on occurrences that relate to the same emotional and intellectual sphere that may have been experienced over many years, causing chronic stress. What matters most is not the occurrence of a negative life event as such, but how a person perceives it. Certain people tend to react to such events with feelings of guilt, hopelessness, shame, hurt and anger. They may have a limited problem-solving capacity and if they also suffer from fatigue or exhaustion, insomnia, or hunger or malnutrition, the onset of the suicidal process may be rapid for people who are susceptible but otherwise not suicidal. A relatively minor additional negative event may then be all it takes to precipitate a suicidal act (see also Chapter 14).

Negative life events

An unexpected change in a person's life situation (an actual or threatened loss, or failure at home or at work) may bring to the fore memories of similar situations and perceptions of injury. This is a clear risk situation for suicide. Several studies have shown that negative life events act both as catalysts in the suicidal process and as factors that precipitate suicide. In a major Finnish study of 1067 suicide victims,[1-3] recent negative life events were found to have occurred in 80% of cases. The most frequent life events were problems at work (experienced by 28%), family discord (23%), somatic illness (22%), financial problems (18%), unemployment (16%), separation (14%), death of a family member (13%) and illness in the family (12%). The women had often experienced more negative life events than the men.

Young people undergo separations more often than their elders and also have more severe problems in relationships with the family, more setbacks in terms of finances, work and unemployment. Among the young, many life events are brought about by the individuals themselves. Among middle-aged and elderly people who commit suicide, on the other hand, somatic morbidity and problems connected with retirement are more prevalent. Life events that act as both acute and chronic stressors in suicide appear to have a cumulative effect.

Suicide rates are elevated among workers in certain occupations – chemists, farmers, police officers, artists, doctors and mental health-care staff.[4] The relatively high propensity of these groups to commit suicide may be the result of complex interaction between stress factors at work, the access to the means of suicide and other risk factors, such as psychiatric and personality disorders.

Actual and threatened losses

Apart from separation from a partner or friend, a separation or loss may involve the loss of possessions, functions or relationships that have afforded security. For some people, when everyday life changes no longer provide a purposeful existence, suicide risk is high. This applies particularly to those who have difficulty in finding a new purpose in everyday life and settling into new routines.[5]

Loss of a significant other

The disappearance of a key person (e.g. a partner, relative, friend, neighbour or a home help (for an elderly or disabled person)) who provided practical help and a boost to the suicidal person's self-image may be a major loss. The frustration is particularly acute for people with marked dependency needs. Goethe, in 'Westöstlicher Divan' has described so aptly this kind of reaction: 'When he keeps my hands full, my self seems important and dear . . . he goes, and instantly I am lost.' ('Wei sie sich an mich verschwendet,/Bin ich mir ein wertes Ich;/Hätte sie sich weggewendet,/ Augenblicks verlör ich mich'). The loss of love, activities, meaningful experiences, financial benefits and status that were associated with the lost person may expose an inner sense of emptiness. With simultaneous frustration of security needs, a high-risk situation may arise. A separation that reminds of similar events in the childhood also implies an elevated suicide risk.

After the death of a parent or spouse, suicide risk rises more among men than women and remains elevated for 4–5 years. After suicide of a close family member, the risk of suicide is elevated for other family members during a grief process that is usually long and difficult.

Loss of a national or cultural affiliation
Suicide rates are elevated among refugees who have not yet adjusted to their new country. Separation from the old culture and the shock of sudden confrontation with the new culture tell part of the story. However, separation from the rest of society that is not the entirely voluntary choice of a group or an individual seems also to boost the suicide risk.[6] This applies to many indigenous ethnic groups, such as the American Indians, the Aborigines, and the Inuit (see also Chapter 12).

Loss of health
Falling ill or suffering a relapse, whether the illness is somatic (see Chapter 11) or mental (e.g. depression or psychosis) or consists in substance abuse (see Chapters 4–9), is experienced as a disappointing and negative life event.[7] A new acute phase of a chronic illness forces the sufferer to learn, once more, to live with the illness. Not all people can cope with such a burden.

Hospitalization
For psychiatric patients and elderly people who are chronically ill, admission to hospital may be perceived as a threat to personal autonomy. The risk of a suicidal act before treatment starts is sometimes high.

Temporary leave from hospital
Temporary leave from hospital after a suicide attempt or in the course of treatment for mental illness, when the patient's suicidal ideation is still pronounced, constitutes a risk situation. Such problems may be particularly severe if the ward staff have fragmented perceptions of the patient. Marked processes that involve group dynamics may begin when the patient is perceived in disparate ways by different members of staff. In such situations, proper suicide-risk assessment must be carried out and the psychodynamics of staff interaction on the ward must be analysed (see also Chapter 15).

Discharge from hospital
Discharge from hospital may also be a risk factor.[8] Both repeated suicide attempts and completed suicides often take place shortly after patients

are discharged. Not only suicide mortality but also the rate of death from other causes is particularly high in the first weeks and months after attempted suicide, and they remain elevated for as much as 1 year afterwards. This is probably due to the lack of properly thought-out rehabilitation and follow-up measures. These measures should be planned well in advance of the patient's discharge in co-operation between the hospital, the family and community service providers (see also Chapter 15).

Others' loss of health or life

Illness, whether sudden or chronic, and death of a family member or significant other is a risk situation. For young women, abortion (whether they have chosen it of their own free will or have been compelled by circumstances to undergo it) may arouse a strong sense of guilt and loss. In some young people not developing into a heterosexual can be perceived traumatically and as a loss.

Loss of employment, study opportunities, home and financial position and fear of change

The loss of one's home, failure in studies, unemployment, financial difficulties and bankruptcy are common negative life events among people who commit suicide.

For some people, a change of workplace and even a return to work, which most people regard as something positive, may be risk factors. These events may remind them of previous unsolved problems at the workplace or of their own inability to cope with the duties concerned.

For sensitive young people, choosing an occupation, education, home and partner may constitute a risk situation. Students embarking on higher education, especially during the first and second year, and conscripts in the armed forces at the start and end of their military service can also experience severe stress. This stress, when combined with psychiatric and psychological risk factors, contributes to the elevated suicide rates in these groups.

Sudden wealth or economical loss, due to bankruptcy, gambling, etc may also involve risk if the person has very low self-esteem and is afraid of not meeting the demands of the new situation.

Relationship problems

Suicide is often immediately preceded by various types of problems in relationships with close family members, friends and colleagues.[9] Loneliness and despondency or depression caused by these problems are exacerbating factors. Spouses who are not supportive and who act as a reminder of parents' negative behaviour are a risk for a suicidal person, who is often engaged in a lifelong quest for love, consolation and a supportive existence.

Change in activities due to public holidays

Fluctuations in suicide rates in connection with all major public holidays have been described in several studies.[10] The phenomenon involves a fall in the incidence of suicidal acts before the holiday and a rise after it. In the West, this pattern is particularly marked at Christmas, New Year, Easter and Whitsun, and in the USA in connection with Independence Day (4 July) and Labor Day. It is strikingly similar for suicide and attempted suicide.

The factors involved may include not only the change in the content of everyday activities but also the disappointment of returning to one's workaday existence, thwarted expectations, cumulative relationship problems and abstinence due to overconsumption of alcoholic beverages during leisure days.

Suicide may take place in connection with a 'red-letter day'. The date may be of particular significance to the person concerned, such as when a family member committed suicide, the person's own birthday or some other emotionally loaded anniversary.

Seasonal patterns, with more suicides during the spring and summer than during the winter, are also characteristic.

Changes in life situation

Changing phases of life
Entering or leaving a phase of development, such as puberty, middle age, the menopause or old age, may be perceived as problematic and constitute a risk situation, possibly owing to the loss of the previous content of life before a new one is found or due to a loss of good relationships.[5] People whose happiness has been based on their youth and success in their career may experience ageing as a loss of the youthful, successful self-image and, as such, and experience ageing as a process damaging to their self-esteem.

Change caused by contravention of law or norms
A legal problem, being caught breaking the law, having one's driving or gun licence confiscated, being exposed as an embezzler, or any other disclosure that arouses shame will elevate the suicide risk.

Change caused by imprisonment
Immediately after going into prison or in periods when new legal problems arise (e.g. new charges being brought, a sentence being modified or an appeal to a higher court being rejected) people are in a suicide-risk situation that is often overlooked. When a prisoner receives news of

illness in the family or the loss of a loved one, or experiences some type of narcissistic injury or rejection, this too is a risk situation for suicide. Otherwise, risk factors for prison inmates do not deviate from those for suicide victims in general. The usual psychiatric, psychosocial, somatic and personality factors, as described previously in this book, apply.[11]

Traumas

Violence, physical and mental abuse

Bullying, victimization and harassment at school or the workplace are risk situations for suicide. Clear risk situations also arise when there are acts or threats of violence against the at risk person or others in his or her surroundings. Traumatic events, such as sexual molestation and assault, rape, and physical and mental abuse, are connected with suicide. The same applies to incest, torture and any occurrence that brings to the fore memories of incest, torture or other traumas.[12]

Childhood traumas, with or without violence or abuse, are often unresolved if the child lived in a dysfunctional family that was incapable of looking after him or her. Suicidal people often come from broken homes or homes in which one or both parents were emotionally disturbed or mentally ill. Depression and/or alcoholism are typical features.

War and natural disasters

Veterans of the Vietnam War have been studied in detail, and the findings show a correlation between their traumatic experience and their suicidality. Their elevated rate of suicidal behaviour applied whether they suffered from post-traumatic stress disorder or not.[13] Natural disasters, such as floods, hurricanes and earthquakes, may also precipitate suicidal ideation and culminate in suicide among victims.[14]

Narcissistic injury

All the life events described above may contribute to a perception of injury and attack on one's self-worth. Of paramount importance is the way in which a suicidal person perceives the negative life event – the loss, change or trauma – and, in particular, whether it induces feelings of helplessness and hopelessness (see Chapter 14). A person's coping strategies and the availability of help (whether others offer it, fail to do so or even show a negative or hostile attitude) are other crucial variables, together with the inborn and acquired vulnerability (see Chapter 2).

References

1. Heikkinen M, Aro H, Lönnqvist J. Recent life events, social support and suicide. *Acta Psychiatr Scand Suppl* 1994;**377:**65–72.

2. Heikkinen ME, Isometsa ET, Aro HM, et al. Age-related variation in recent life events preceding suicide. *J Nerv Ment Dis* 1995;**183:**325–331.

3. Isometsa E, Heikkinen M, Henriksson M, et al. Recent life events and completed suicide in bipolar affective disorder. A comparison with major depressive suicides. *J Affect Disord* 1995;**33:**99–106.

4. Boxer PA, Burnett C, Swanson N. Suicide and occupation: a review of the literature. *J Occup Environ Med* 1995;**37:**442–452.

5. Rich C, Warsradt G, Nemiroff R, et al. Suicide, stressors, and the life cycle. *Am J Psychiatry* 1991;**148:**524–527.

6. Lester D. Native American suicide rates, acculturation stress and traditional integration. *Psychol Rep* 1999;**84:**398.

7. Haste F, Charlton J, Jenkins R. Potential for suicide prevention in primary care? An analysis of factors associated with suicide. *Br J Gen Prac* 1998;**48:**1759–1763.

8. Holley HL, Fick G, Love EJ. Suicide following an inpatient hospitalization for a suicide attempt: a Canadian follow-up study. *Soc Psychiatry Epidemiol* 1998;**33:**543–551.

9. Maris RW. Social and familial risk factors in suicidal behaviour. *Psychiatr Clin North Am* 1997;**20:**519–550.

10. Jessen G, Jensen B. Postponed suicide death? Suicides around birthdays and major public holidays. *Suicide Life Threat Behav* 1999;**29:**272–283.

11. Hayes LM. Jail suicide and the need for debriefing. *Crisis* 1997;**18:**150–151.

12. Ferrada-Noli M, Asberg M, Ormstad K. Suicidal behaviour after severe trauma Part 2. The association between methods of torture and of suicidal ideation in posttraumatic stress disorder. *J Trauma Stress* 1998;**11:**113–124.

13. Bullman TA, Kang HK. Posttraumatic stress disorder and the risk of traumatic deaths among Vietnam veterans. *J Nerv Ment Dis* 1994;**182:**604–610.

14. Krug EG, Kresnow M, Peddicord JP, et al. Suicide after natural disasters. *N Engl J Med* 1998;**338:**373–378.

14
Suicidal people's experiences of negative life events

Danuta Wasserman

This chapter presents the emotional experiences of suicidal people when negative life events, as described in Chapter 13, push them to suicide.

Early years leave their mark

Suicidal people's attitudes towards and reactions to current negative life events must be seen in the light of the frustration of their fundamental needs. Their needs – to be seen, loved and acknowledged – are not only being frustrated in the current situation but have also been since early childhood.[1]

Suicidal people's relationships, past and present, have often been characterized by humiliation, narcissistic injury and rejection. Similarly, their current emotional and cognitive perceptions and reactions are usually loaded with memories and feelings associated with early object losses and a negative emotional climate in the family home. Their parents may have been strict, quick to punish and lacking in empathy, or characteristically indifferent or overprotective, overstepping the normal limits of the parental role and failing to respond to the child's needs. With a lack of good examples of communication skills and speech and behavior during childhood and with suicidal behaviour experienced as a model in the family home, suicidal people tend to be influenced towards choosing self-destructive acts as a way out when negative life events once more bring their lack of self-confirmation to the fore.[2]

Lack of self-love

Much has been written about narcissism among suicidal people, and there are numerous interpretations of the Narkissos myth. For people who are close to suicide, however, the problem is their lack of self-love rather than any exaggerated love of self. What they experience is a thirst for confirmation from others, and they are devastated by its absence.

Suicidal people long for love, intimacy and appreciation. Their hunger to satisfy these needs is often masked by their efforts that are aimed at concealing it. This behaviour may be misinterpreted by others as showing that they are provocative, self-sufficient, cold and rejecting. Close up, however, the thinness and fragility of the deeply distressed and dissatisfied suicidal person's psychological defence mechanisms become apparent.[3]

Shame

Morbid shame about not being loved and appreciated and about being unable to live up to the high ideals and standards that suicidal people have usually imposed on themselves is common. They feel inferior, of little worth, weak and uncertain, while at the same time dreaming of being loved, cherished and valued. Their dream of strength and security is thwarted to the utmost by negative life events. Shame permeates their personality, and arises when their 'shortcomings' are laid bare by a situation of loss and/or offence.[4]

However, suicidal people may be tormented by shame even when they are in fact loved, successful and good at what they do. They are constantly plagued by an innermost feeling, which stems from their early years, that no one can love them since what is below the surface is so terrible. They cannot enjoy their successes. Their feelings that the acknowledgement that they receive is given for something that they have not deserved, and that they have in fact deceived others, reinforces their shame.

The shame requires them to become different, to 'reinvent' themselves, and if this proves impossible, suicidal impulses become stronger. A desperate urge to wipe out a part of oneself that is perceived as bad can lead to suicidal acts.[5]

Narcissistic injury

Grave injury to the self-respect often precipitate suicidal behaviours. Suicidal persons have a disastrous propensity and talent for provoking constant repetitions of various types of injury or offence. Not infrequently, these appear to confirm that they are not loved, needed or wanted. Many suicidal people are, moreover, so sensitive as to take offence in situations that would never be perceived as hurtful by other people. This tendency may sometimes be so marked that a long series of actual or imaginary offences can eventually be interpreted as a coherent pattern, and suicidal people therefore adopt a paranoid attitude towards others. The narcissistic injury does not result in grief and working through, but in bitterness, longing after revenge and furious outbursts, with self-destructive acts as a result.

This does not exclude the possibility that suicidal people may, in fact, be ill-treated by others, including health-care staff. This is blamed on the individuals' tendency to take offence, which in turn makes them even more implacable and filled with resignation and hate.[5]

Anger and rage

The step from narcissistic injury and shame to anger and rage is a very short one.[6] Suicidal situations are precipitated when people feel that they have been 'revealed' and their innermost beings have been laid bare. This exposure may take place with the disappearance of, for example, a much-loved partner who has contributed greatly to the suicidal person's self-confidence, the caring parent who has looked after the schizophrenic boy all his life, wealth or one's beloved country, together with the security that such people, circumstances and things provided. Anger and rage is close when real-life circumstances that have held at bay the undesired self-image no longer exist, since the undesired self-image cannot be fended off solely by means of fantasies. If a person's affect-neutralizing ability is poor, losses and offences are perceived as being so severe, injurious and insurmountable that the longing to die can seem the only way out.

Guilt

Guilt is another feeling that dominates suicidal people's consciousness.[7,8] High self-ideals and strict, almost archaic and rigid moral norms contribute to self-reproach, which readily arises when negative life events occur. The next step easily leads to anxiety and guilt about not succeeding, in contrast to others. The sense of guilt may grow strong and prompt efforts to make amends that may sometimes be directly contrary to the suicidal person's own interests and instinct of self-preservation. A vicious circle may arise when others, instead of being grateful as the suicidal person expects, call this behaviour in question, are surprised or show a non-committal attitude.

Guilt can also be experienced as a result of unconscious or conscious hostile or revenge feelings towards an 'ambivalent' (loved and at the same time hated) lost object.[9]

Guilt caused by hatred of parents or spouse may make a person feel so wicked that suicide may present itself as a deserved punishment. Feelings of guilt and shame also reinforce negative self-perception, with the result that suicide is chosen as a means of escape from this painful awareness.

Despair and hopelessness

Despair and hopelessness concerning the future are other affective states that often present in suicidal persons when they experience losses, traumas and other major life changes (see Chapter 13). Fantasies of rebirth or reunion with a lost object through suicide can be strong, along with ideas of worthlessness.[10,11]

Paradoxical behaviour

Suicidal people's behaviour may sometimes be paradoxical, and it is not unusual for this behaviour to bring about negative life events. A suicidal person may have a fear that his or her dependence on confirmation from others, his or her innermost sense of worthlessness and his or her shame about being abandoned will be discovered; therefore, the suicidal person may compensate by deluding family members and hospital staff into a false sense of security and may succeed in convincing these people that he or she can manage without their help while at the same time feeling unable to do so. Through rejection of people whom he or she loves or needs, a suicidal person may create an illusion of control over an inter-personal relationship.[12]

To avoid disclosure and the need to feel shame for the 'unworthiness' that suicidal people perceive inside themselves, they mask their vulnerability with such defences as fantasies of greatness and emphasis on their independence and invulnerability, despite their great dependency and vulnerability.[5]

Denial of real-life circumstances, which results in brutal confrontations that boost the risk of suicide, is another means of self-defence against their own vulnerability. By failing to re-examine their own emotional and cognitive perceptions, suicidal people bring ruin on themselves and put their own lives at stake.

Suicidal people's ambivalence can be used to save their lives, not to hasten death

But what guilt, shame or hurt can be so great as to make people choose death? There is no universal answer to this question, since individual experience cannot be transmitted from one person to another, or from one person to a group. No generalizations can be made. However, a suicidal person is almost always ambivalent about the choice between life and death to the very last. Ambivalent feelings are mixed feelings. Paralysing doubt alternates with thoughts cast hither and thither, resignation, misgivings and cancellations. Tunnel vision, which restricts and distorts perceptions, is typical in suicidal individuals (see also Chapter 2).

There is a difference between the healthy ambivalence that is a basic human emotion, the healthy doubt that leads us forward, and the pathological ambivalence that paralyses a person. This pathological ambivalence is a matter of inadequate integration of different affects and their cognitive and intellectual contents. Among suicidal people, good and evil identification objects, the wish to live and the wish to die, a need to be extremely dependent and a need to be extremely independent, and love and hate often coexist and compete with each other. They do not readily blend, become integrated and serve as guidance in how to live a more harmonious life. Even minor negative life events and instances of inadequate support from family and friends may therefore be fatal for some suicidal people.

It is essential to listen and respond to the shame, hurt and guilt expressed by people who have severe suicidal ideation, referred to suicide plans or attempted suicide, as well as by people who have had relatives who have such a history. By listening, one may help to detect the ambivalence that is always present in those who are contemplating taking their own lives. This ambivalence can be used to arrest the negative development of the suicidal process and prevent a premature and unnecessary death.[5,13]

If we are 'deaf' to the suicidal communication and vulnerability of those who are close to suicide, their self-destruction may ensue.

References

1. Shneidman ES. The suicidal mind. Oxford University Press. New York; 1996.

2. Apter A, Plutchik R, Sevy S, et al. Defense mechanisms in risk of suicide and risk of violence. *Am J Psychiatry* 1989;**146:**1027–1031

3. Leenaars A, Lester D. Suicide and the unconscious. Northvale, NJ, USA: J Aronson; 1996.

4. Kernberg O. Diagnosis and clinical management of suicidal potential in borderline patients: the borderline patient, vol 2. Hillsdale NJ, USA: Analytic Press; 1987.

5. Wolk-Wasserman D. Attempted suicide: the patient's family, social network and therapy (Doctoral Dissertation). Stockholm: Karolinska Institute; 1986.

6. Hendin H. The psychodynamics of suicide with particular reference to the young. *Am J Psychiatry* 1991;**148:**1150–1158.

7. Hendin H, Haas A. Suicide and guilt as manifestations of PTSD in Vietnam combat veterans. *Am J Psychiatry* 1991;**148:**586–591.

8. Hendin H. The psychodynamics of suicide. *J Nerv Ment Dis* 1963;**136:**236–244.

9. Freud S. Mourning and melancholia. In: Strachey J (ed). The standard edition of the complete psychological works of Sigmund Freud, volume XIV. London: Hogarth Press; 1957:243–258.

10. Maltsberger JT, Bui DH. The devices of suicide: revenge, riddance, and rebirth. *Int Rev Psychoanal* 1980;**7:**61–72

11. Maltsberger JT, Bui DH. The psychological vulnerability to suicide.

In: Jacobs D, Brown H (eds). Suicide: understanding and responding. Madison CT, USA: International Universities Press; 1989;59–72.

12. Lifton R. Suicide. In: Jacobs D, Brown H (eds). Suicide: understanding and responding. Madi-son CT, USA: International Universities Press; 1989;459–469.

13. Duilt RA, Michaels R. Psychodynamics and suicide. In: Jacobs D (ed). Suicide and clinical practice. Washington, DC: American Psychiatric Press; 1990:44–53.

15

Attempted suicide as a risk factor for suicide: treatment and follow-up

Nils Retterstøl and Lars Mehlum

Introduction

Owing to the lack of national and international epidemiological routine data on attempted suicide (parasuicide) our knowledge about the magnitude of this problem is largely based on monitoring studies from defined catchment areas and on cross-sectional self-report studies. According to the World Health Organization (WHO) European multicentre study on parasuicide[1] the male parasuicide rate varied from 45 to 314 per 100,000 of the population from the lowest to the highest level among the 13 participating countries. The female parasuicide rate ranged from 69 to 462 per 100,000 of the population. In all countries except Finland parasuicide was more common in females than in males; the female–male ratio generally varied from 1.5:1 to 3:1. For children and adolescents, parasuicide seems to be much more common in females than in males. The parasuicide rate seems to be higher in younger age groups than in older age groups. We should, however, remember that monitoring studies such as the WHO study include only parasuicides that come to the attention of the health service; these cases may well be only the tip of the iceberg, particularly in the younger age groups. A conservative estimate would indicate that attempted suicide is at least 10 times more common than completed suicide.

Predictors for completed suicide

Attempted suicide is the strongest and probably the most universal of all known predictors of suicide. According to research, approximately 10% of those who have been admitted to psychiatric treatment after a suicide attempt will eventually commit suicide. An additional 10–50%, depending on population characteristics, will repeat their suicide attempts. Within the group of suicide attempters the following characteristics seem to indicate a higher risk of later suicide:[2-5]

- male sex;
- age above 45 years;
- separated, divorced or widowed status;
- unemployment or old age retirement;
- chronic somatic illness;
- major psychiatric disorder;
- personality disorder;
- alcohol or other substance use disorder;
- the use of violent methods for suicide; and
- the leaving of a suicide note.

Affective disorders such as major depression, schizophrenia, certain personality disorders and substance use disorders are all well documented predictors for suicide. Severe anxiety disorders such as panic disorder may also lead to an increased risk of suicide.

The danger of completed suicide is generally greatest in the first year (and particularly in the first 3 months) after the suicide attempt.[2-5] The patient is often labile and vulnerable to stress during this period and needs adequate protection and support. This support should be sustained throughout the first year after the suicidal crisis.

Despite the evident danger of suicide, it is important to remember that 90% of suicide attempters survive. According to follow-up studies many patients report their suicidal attempts as being the major reason for them receiving help or coming under psychiatric treatment.[4] Therefore, in many cases the suicide attempt should be regarded as a golden opportunity for patients, in collaboration with clinicians, to solve problems that would otherwise not be identified or available for treatment.

Clinical challenges

When working with suicide attempters, clinicians are faced with three central challenges:

- to protect the patient against repetition of attempted suicide and against suicide or irreversible injury;
- to reduce the patient's profound feeling of hopelessness; and
- to elevate the patient's subjective experience of quality of life.

Patients who have attempted suicide often require treatment in an emergency room and then need to be observed for the next 1–3 days in an acute medical ward. A psychiatric examination, in which an adequate history is taken and the suicide intent and the danger of suicide is evaluated, should be conducted as early as possible during this early treatment phase and in any event before the patient is discharged from hospital. The psychiatric consultation should provide information that is necessary for treatment planning, and it should also serve as a clinical intervention focusing on the patient's most critical problems and psychological needs. To establish a therapeutic alliance is of utmost importance for the prospects of successful treatment of patients in suicidal crises. While patients must get the opportunity to recover from their medical condition (e.g. the intoxication) and to rest in an atmosphere of kindness and reassurance, most patients also need to give verbal expression to their problems and emotions, with the therapist's help. Some of these emotions may be of such a nature as to easily evoke countertransference reactions in the therapist[6] (the arousal of the therapist's own repressed feelings through identification with the patient's experiences and problems or through a response in kind to the patient's expressions of love or hostility toward him or her), in which case this must be dealt with properly through professional supervision (see also Chapter 17). The therapist needs to demonstrate acceptance of the patient but not necessarily of the suicidal behaviour and to discuss problem-solving strategies other than suicide. Most patients are initially in a state of emotional turmoil and chaos and need help to get a better understanding of what has happened to them and why.

After the initial medical treatment is completed, some patients can be discharged and followed up on an out-patient basis. In such cases it is important to involve the patient's family, if at all possible, in order to organize protective measures, motivate for treatment, increase the patient's compliance and to give emotional support. The family must be given proper information (provided that the patient does not object to this). If the patient's life is in imminent danger it may be necessary to breach confidentiality.

Hospital treatment

The presence of one or more of the following characteristics indicates that the patient should be transferred without delay for psychiatric in-patient treatment:

- suicide attempts made with a high degree of suicidal intent;
- a continued wish or plan for suicide;
- symptoms of severe mental disorder, such as major depression or psychosis, and alcohol or other substance misuse/use disorder;
- poor impulse control or weak barriers against suicide;
- poor social support; and
- recent severe social stressors, loss or emotional trauma.

Sometimes the patient refuses to be hospitalized. If in such cases there is imminent danger to the patient's life, involuntary commitment is often necessary.

When the patient is transferred to a psychiatric hospital there is a need to promote the establishment of a new therapeutic alliance through measures mentioned above. A clinical re-evaluation should be conducted immediately and, depending on the results, all necessary safety measures should be undertaken to place the patient in a secure room with safety windows and to remove the patient's belt, razors and other dangerous objects. Some patients must be observed continuously; in any case frequent observations are needed. Control measures have the potential of threatening the patient's personal integrity and should therefore be implemented with care and respect. Before free exit or home leave is permitted careful evaluation must be performed and the patient's family should be informed. In order to reduce the need of control measures over prolonged periods of time the staff may ask the patient to sign or to verbally agree to a 'no suicide' contract, in which the patient agrees not to harm himself or herself for a specific period of time and to contact the staff if his or her feelings or the situation changes.[7] To a certain extent the patient's impulse control can be strengthened, symptoms alleviated and the tendency of substance abuse reduced through effective use of antidepressant or antipsychotic agents (or both). If a patient who has signs of major depression does not respond to antidepressants or if it is too risky to wait for several weeks for the antidepressants to become effective, a trial of electroconvulsive therapy may be appropriate.

Elderly patients

Elderly patients admitted after suicide attempts often suffer from major depression, which is frequently related to social isolation or a sense of worthlessness linked to a reduced physical or mental capability.[8] Somatic illness or polypharmacy may give rise to depression or pharmacological side effects. Existential problems must be dealt with psychotherapeutically and through social work or family interventions, and somatic problems must be diagnosed and treated. In the short term it is seldom possible to invoke radical changes for the better in the patient's life. However, even minor changes may have the potential of reducing the patient's feeling of hopelessness; this is an important objective in all clinical interventions with suicidal patients.

The suicide rate in single men over 80 years of age is particularly high. The mortality from suicide increases with social isolation and particularly after loss of a spouse. Previous suicide attempts, particularly violent suicide attempts, in elderly men and women generally imply a much higher risk of subsequent successful completion of suicide than they do in young people.

Young suicide attempters

In young suicide attempters, depression is often a prominent clinical feature. Parents and other family members must be involved in the process of treatment unless there is a special reason to avoid this (e.g. the patient having been sexually abused by one of the parents). Personality disorders are frequently a part of the clinical picture in young suicide attempters.[9] Some of them have developed a pattern of chronic suicidal behaviour, which may be hard to treat effectively. Such cases should be referred for specialized psychiatric treatment, such as dialectic behavioural therapy,[10] after the acute crisis has subsided. Young females who have developed suicidal feelings seem generally to possess better help-seeking skills and to be more easily available for assessment and treatment than young males. Many suicidal young males are characterized by anger or other problems which affect regulation, antisocial behaviour and denial of depression and may thus be less accessible for clinical intervention.

Out-patient treatment

The patient's discharge from hospital should be carefully planned and a suitable after-care treatment programme organized. Depending on the clinical picture there may be a need for follow-up of medication, referral for alcohol or drug rehabilitation, and individual or family therapy. Some patients can rely on their family doctor to co-ordinate the various treatment components. In many cases, however, patients have difficulties seeking help or complying with the treatment that is offered to them. This calls for an active and rehabilitative approach from the therapist's side. In some agencies organized teams follow up suicide attempters through home visits and practical and problem-solving-oriented assistance during the first few weeks after discharge from hospital. It is highly important to create a continuous chain of care, beginning with the emergency phase of the treatment, continuing with hospital treatment and leading eventually to some form of after-care programme.

Longitudinal studies have shown that patients treated for suicide attempts run a particularly high risk of completed suicide during the first year after discharge.[2-5] In many cases the patient should remain in out-patient treatment throughout this first year. The duration of such follow-up treatment must, however, be tailored to the individual patient's needs and can often be gradually attenuated and finally terminated. Such measures have resulted in a reduction of drop-out rates and promising results regarding the tendency of the patient to repeat the suicidal behaviour. There is, however, still a lack of randomized trials that have compared the efficacy of different psychosocial and pharmacological treatment protocols. In a systematic review of 20 trials,[11] the following protocols resulted in reduced repetition of deliberate self harm:

- problem solving therapy;
- the provision of an emergency contact card in addition to standard care;
- trials of intensive after-care plus outreach;
- dialectical behaviour therapy; and
- the administration of depot flupenthixol.

Future research will, it is hoped, give better directions about which type of therapy and in which combinations is optimal for individual patients.

Case history

A 25-year-old woman with emotionally and economically deprived background was engaged to be married, but at the last moment the engagement was called off. Gravely disappointed she moved abroad and found herself a job in a nursing home. Soon afterwards she developed anxiety symptoms and had persecutory delusions whereby she felt that her colleagues and her landlord wanted to harm her. Despite an increasing fear that she would be killed, she did not reveal these problems to anybody and did not seek help.

Finally, she decided to return home and left by train, where she suddenly was overwhelmed by the impression that the whole train was full of persecutors. In panic she jumped from the train window, which resulted in serious injuries and fractures. Naturally she was hospitalized and after completion of her surgical treatment she was transferred to a psychiatric ward.

After 1 month of treatment with neuroleptics and supportive psychotherapy she was discharged and included in a systematic after-care programme. Soon, she was able to seek new employment. Her treatment continued for 2 years and was supervised by the psychiatric out-patient department in close collaboration with the local doctor and district nurse.

Currently, 25 years later, she lives autonomously and is self-supporting with a job as an assistant nurse. She has a limited but nourishing social network in her local community. She is not married and has no children but participates in a couple of local women's clubs. She has had no more psychotic episodes or suicide attempts. The suicide attempt seems in this case to have served as a trigger for the patient to come under psychiatric treatment for a severe psychotic disorder, and systematic after-care has probably given a more favourable clinical course and outcome and has probably also prevented repeated suicidal behaviour.

References

1. Schmidtke A, Bille-Brahe U, DeLeo D, et al. Attempted suicide in Europe: rates, trends and sociodemographic characteristics of suicide attempters during the period 1989–92. Results of the WHO/EURO Multicentre Study on Parasuicide. *Acta Psychiatr Scand* 1996;**93:**327–338.

2. Dahlgren KG. Attempted suicide: 35 years afterwards. *Suicide Life Threat Behav* 1977;**7:**75–79.

3. Ekeberg Ø, Ellingsen Ø, Jacobsen D. Suicide and other causes of death in a five-year follow-up period of patients treated for self-poisoning in Oslo. *Acta Psychiatr Scand* 1991;**83:**432–437.

4. Retterstøl N. Long-term prognosis after attempted suicide. Thomas, Springfield. 1970.

5. Hawton K, Fagg J. Suicide and other causes of death, following attempted suicide. *Br J Psychiatry* 1988;**152:**359–366.

6. Maltsberger JT, Buie DH. Countertransference hate in the treatment of suicidal patients. *Arch Gen Psychiatry* 1974;**30:**625–633.

7. Stanford EJ, Goetz RR, Bloom JD. The no harm contract in emergency assessment of suicidal risk. *J Clin Psychiatry* 1994;**55:**344–348.

8. Osgood NJ, Thielman S. Geriatric suicidal behavior: assessment and treatment. In: Blumenthal SJ, Kupfer DJ (eds). Suicide over the life cycle: risk factors, assessment, and treatment of suicidal patients. Washington: American Psychiatric Press; 1990;341–379.

9. Mehlum L, Friis S, Vaglum P, Karterud S. The longitudinal pattern of suicidal behaviour in borderline personality disorder: a prospective follow-up study. *Acta Psychiatr Scand* 1994;**90:** 124–130.

10. Linehan MM, Armstrong HE, Suarez A, et al. Cognitive–behavioral treatment for chronically parasuicidal borderline patients. *Arch Gen Psychiatry* 1991;**48:**1060–1064.

11. Hawton K, Arensman E, Townsend E, et al. Deliberate self harm: systematic review of efficacy of psychosocial and pharmacological treatments in preventing repetition. *BMJ* 1998; **317:**441–447.

16
Suicide risk assessment

Danuta Wasserman

Systematic clinical assessment of suicide risk

Suicide risk assessment is the most difficult kind of assessment in psy-chiatric practice, since it is about life and death and arouses fear in doc-tors themselves. Doctors need not – and cannot – assume responsibility for the life of a suicidal patient but, on the other hand, they must put their knowledge into practice in an optimal way with the goal of preventing a threatening suicide.

Many suicidal patients, like other psychiatric patients, hesitate to con-sult a psychiatrist for as long as possible. Not infrequently, they finally do so after repeated urging from family members, friends or colleagues. It is therefore essential to give such patients ample time and attention. Assessment of suicide risk touches on patients' most pressing problems, including their reflections on life and death. It includes the causes of their suicidality and their future prospects. It also encompasses what suicidal patients have themselves done to solve their problems, and their expec-tations of care.[1]

Suicide risk assessment should take place on several levels and relate to the patient, his or her families and social networks and also to the availability of treatment, rehabilitation and prevention resources in the community. Assessing risk involves considering factors that exacerbate and factors that hinder the development of the suicidal process such as:

- suicidal intention;
- previous psychiatric disorders and suicidal behaviour;
- suicide in the family or acquaintances (suicide models); and
- the patient's suicidal communication.

Assessment of the nature of family members, friends and networks is also vital. If, for example, there are no negative life events and the family is supportive, suicide risk does not necessarily arise.

In addition to a clinical interview, one may use the instruments suggested in Chapter 18, which form part of various appraisal scales, to evaluate suicide risk. The questions posed must feel natural both to the patient and to the doctor (see also Chapter 17).

The suicidal process

Suicide risk is a crescendo phenomenon. Movement from sporadic thoughts of death to more frequent suicide wishes or from diffuse suicide plans to schemes that include detailed choices of method and place in the near future indicate there is a rising scale of suicide risk in the suicidal process. Advanced suicide plans or actual attempts with a high intentionality and pronounced anxiety[2] as well as with active methods, indicate high suicide risk. People who have easily aroused feelings of hopelessness, suicidal ideation and a history of previous suicide attempts, and also those who have models in the form of family members or acquaintances who have attempted or committed suicide, make up a clear group in terms of long-term risk of suicidal behaviour[3] (see also Chapter 2).

In some cases the above described crescendo phenomenon can be repeated during the suicidal patient's life (a cyclical course); for example, a suicide attempt can be performed by a young female or male at the age of 15 or 16 and be repeated when they are 24 or 30, or later on in their lives.

In assessing suicide risk, one must ask questions and explore the answers to questions such as: What does life mean to this person? Is there anything that appeals to him or her? What is about to happen in the patient's life, over the next 24 hours or the month ahead? If he or she invariably looks on the dark side and has no plans for the future or supportive resources – family, friends or work – the risk of suicide is high.

Suicidal communication

Suicidal communication may range from no hint of suicidal intent or just the occasional expression of suicidal intent in upsetting situations – sometimes under the influence of alcohol, and indicating little or no risk of suicide – to suicidal statements of intent with a blend of seriousness and denial that distinctly alarms other people and indicates medium to high risk. Repeated, clear verbal expression of serious suicidal thoughts and suicide plans without being under the influence of alcohol or a quarrel indicates a high suicide risk.

Relationships

Suicide risk is low if the patient has good relationships with relatives or friends who are ready to help in times of need. Such relationships imply prospects of successfully working through the kinds of problems that trigger the suicidal situation. On the other hand, suicide risk is elevated if the patient's relationships are characterized by ambiguous communication, ambivalence and aggressiveness, and if close relatives and friends have long since given up hope of cohabiting or socializing with him or her. In this situation, it is important to assess whether the family and closest friends can serve as support for the suicidal person in the treatment, or whether the family or social network itself needs support or treatment.

Sometimes risk is difficult to assess if there are frequent separations from and reconciliations with one and the same partner, or if there are relationships that undergo constant ups and downs, with growing social problems. If, in such a situation, relationships are definitively broken off, suicide risk is high.

Psychosocial situation

Male, elderly, divorced, single or unemployed people (see also Chapter 12) who have simultaneous alcohol abuse, mental illness or personality disorder and who experience adverse life events are at high risk of suicide if they have previously entertained serious suicide plans or attempted suicide.

Mental illnesses and personality disorders

A renewed bout of depression, manic–depressive illness or other psychosis when negative life events are present and the suicidal person has begun resorting to alcohol may push him or her rapidly from a group characterized by low or medium to high suicide risk into a very high-risk group.[4,5] If this happens, immediate intervention by the family and the health-care services is required.

However, when a patient is reluctant to undergo treatment, even very experienced health-care staff may unfortunately shy away from compulsory treatment or hospitalisation due to an exaggerated fear of violating the patient's integrity.

Patients who can cope with their life situation without exposing themselves to undue stress and strain and who can manage the treatment of their basic illnesses while receiving support from their family or friends do not necessarily have a high suicide risk, although more or less intense suicidal ideation is constantly present. For these people, especially those with dysthymic personality traits and protracted, chronic depression, suicidal ideation is one way of relating to life.

It is sometimes difficult to assess suicide risk in patients with dysthymia or brain damage whose suicidal process is chronic. It can also be difficult to assess suicide risk in immature, impulsive, or violent young people with a prepondency to act out their fantasies.[6]

In Chapters 4–10 and 13 more details can be found about the mental illnesses and personality types that contribute to suicide risk in the event of an unfavourable social situation and of definitive, sudden losses and narcissistic injuries.

Substance abuse

Abuse of alcohol or narcotics in conjunction with other psychiatric morbidity, risk of social exclusion and definitive, sudden losses or narcissistic injuries imply a high suicide risk (see Chapter 5). The risk is often reduced by immediate hospitalization and by starting rehabilitation and treatment of the abuse and the underlying psychiatric morbidity simultaneously.

Somatic illness

Somatic illnesses and situations that place people in the risk zone for suicide are described in Chapter 11. The risk of suicide may be high in people suffering from disabling, painful or terminal illnesses who simultaneously develop depression and experience sudden losses or narcissistic injuries in the absence of good support from the family and adequate pain relief and proper nursing. Illnesses in organs of symbolic importance to the individual, such as breasts to a woman or genital organs to both sexes, may contribute to an elevated suicide risk when other risk factors are also present.

Suicide risk assessment after suicide attempts

In a regressed state (after attempting suicide) suicidal patients' psychological defence mechanisms are weakened. When they regain consciousness after attempting suicide, patients are usually in a state of profound despair and feel ashamed, although they are also often highly relieved to be alive still and wish to be helped. It is therefore much easier at this time to explore their affective state and problems. But in a few hours patients may rapidly 'close up' again and deny their need of help. It is therefore essential to try to fit the suicide-risk assessment into a therapeutic 'window of opportunity', when patients have neither regressed too far nor once again lost contact with their desperation and distanced themselves from the need for professional help and lost motivation for treatment.[7]

Many people repeat their suicide attempts, or commit suicide, very soon after being discharged from hospital. This is partly due to poor treatment compliance, which in turn could be the result of poorly 'timed' suicide-risk assessment.[8,9] The doctor should ensure not only that the patient is given the name of the person responsible for follow-up and an appointment for an initial return visit but also that contact with the patient has taken place.

Suicide risk assessment before temporary discharge
Striking the right balance between keeping suicidal patients in hospital too long and discharging them too early is not easy. Temporary discharge – a day or weekend out – may be a good test of the suicidal patient's ability to cope with reality. Before every temporary discharge, the doctor needs to get in touch with the patient's relatives and to be in a position to judge whether there are supportive factors in the patient's surroundings or whether the problems are still so severe as to entail a risk of suicide.[3]

Assessment for the purpose of discharge, whether temporary or permanent, is paramount since several surveys from various countries show that many patients take their lives shortly after leaving psychiatric hospital (see also Chapter 15).

Previous psychiatric care and the patient's attitude towards care

Suicide risk is high if a patient has previously been admitted to in-patient psychiatric care for mental illness or a suicide attempt and has an ambivalent or even hostile attitude towards care services. The same is true if such a patient has declined or broken off treatment or failed to understand the purpose of undergoing treatment at all. Suicide risk is also exacerbated when psychiatric patients relapse (recurrent disease) due to psychological distress or a critical change in their life, and when they feel at the same time that no one understands them, or they experience paranoid ideation and think that they are being persecuted.

It is sometimes difficult to assess suicide risk in patients who show rapid swings between a positive and perhaps a flattering attitude towards staff and a negative attitude, with open hostility and rejection of the care offered. Elevated suicide risk is indicated by previous psychiatric care without mutual trust between the patient and the staff who provided the care and by swings between negative and positive attitudes to the doctor in charge and care services in general. If, on the other hand, the patient has shown appreciation of care received previously and has expressed confidence in the staff providing the treatment, and has the same attitude in the current situation, suicide risk is low.

Respect for suicidal patients' wishes

Few people commit suicide after mature and balanced consideration. Most patients show distinct psychiatric conditions or psychological distress and are too regressive in their conceptual world with its restricted cognition ('tunnel vision') to be capable of exerting responsibility for themselves at the moment when suicidal ideation is very strong and suicide plans are in the forefront of their minds. Therefore, it is important not only to emphasize patients' responsibility for their own lives, but also to be prepared to assume responsibility and to initiate supportive measures (and sometimes to impose restrictions, including involving compulsory institutional care).

It is important for doctors to have a sense of commitment to their patients and to speak frankly to them and their families. It is also essential for the doctor to point out that, as a professional, he or she is aware that the desire to commit suicide is often ambivalent in nature and, in most cases, disappears when the problems fade away and the psychiatric illness is treated.

Assuming professional responsibility

To assess suicide risk properly, it is vital for doctors to be aware of their own psychological functioning and of how far they themselves fear suicidal fantasies, death, weakness and abandonment.[10] This awareness may be helpful, not only in attempts to convince patients of the value of life, but also in listening to patients' arguments about their reasons for choosing death. Suicidal patients should, in the assessment of suicide risk, be allowed to describe and contemplate their own problems with respect to life, death and suicide, without being made to feel guilty or ashamed. A patient should not feel that such matters are taboo in his or her talks with doctors who assess suicide risk. This kind of open attitude on the doctor's part often relieves the patient's tension and may even reduce suicide risk.

Reducing and gauging risk of suicide

In assessing suicide risk, the doctor must be prepared to take steps that immediately reduce the suicide risk.[11] These steps are often of a psychiatric, psychological and psychosocial nature, including (in certain cases) immediate commitment to hospital. It is important to remember that suicide risk is always changing: today it is different from yesterday and tomorrow it will be different from today. It is therefore vital to monitor patients and their families in order to be able to assess the development of the suicidal process again, in a clinically sensitive way. Various scales may then be helpful (see Chapter 18), especially those designed for self-appraisal, which can arouse the patient's curiosity and bring an element of activity into the treatment. Patients can see concrete results by being able, for example, to monitor their own scores and thus feeling as if they are taking their destiny into their own hands. These scales may also be useful for patients who have a poor communicative capacity or are reluctant to confide in the doctor or care staff.

After completion of suicide risk assessment

Suicide risk assessment should culminate in a conclusion as to whether the risk is low, high or difficult to assess. In the concluding discussion with the doctor, patients should be asked whether there are any other matters that the doctor has omitted to ask about, whether the patient received answers to their own questions, and whether the family can be contacted.

Once a suicide risk assessment has been completed, it is vital to take active steps to transfer the patient to the relevant facilities to receive the further care that is deemed appropriate. The relatives, when the patient's consent is given, should be informed of the procedure and whom to contact if they need to. Similarly, they should be told whom to contact if the patient breaks off treatment.

References

1. Leenaars AA. Clinical evaluation of suicide risk. *Psychiatry Clin Neurosci* 1995;**49(Suppl 1):** S61–S68.

2. Fawcett J, Scheftner WA, Fogg L, et al. Time-related predictors of suicide in major affective disorder. *Am J Psychiatry* 1990;**147:** 1189–1194.

3. Botsis AJ. Suicidal behavior: risk and protective factors. Amsterdam: Elsevier Science; 1997:129–143.

4. Hall RC, Platt DE, Hall RC. Suicide risk assessment: a review of risk factors for suicide in 100 patients who made severe suicide attempts. Evaluation of suicide risk in a time of managed care. *Psychosomatics* 1999;**40:** 18–27.

5. Hawton K. Assessment of suicide risk. *Br J Psychiatry* 1987;**150:** 145–153.

6. Feinstein R, Plutchik R. Violence and suicide risk assessment in

the psychiatric emergency room. *Compr Psychiatry* 1990;**31:** 337–343.

7. Wolk-Wasserman D. The intensive care unit and the suicide attempt patient. *Acta Psychiatr Scand* 1985;**71:** 581–595.

8. Sonneck G, Sjogren C. Contribution to suicide risk assessment II. on the practice of suicide risk assessment. *Crisis* 1990;**11:** 34–36.

9. Tredget J. Suicide risk assessment and the use of patient contracts. *Nurs Times* 1999;**95:** 50–51.

10. Tabachnik N. Countertransference crises in suicidal attempts. *Arch Gen Psychiatry* 1961; **4:**64–70.

11. Morriss R, Gask L, Battersby L, et al. Teaching front-line health and voluntary workers to assess and manage suicidal patients. *J Affect Disord* 1999;**52:**77–83.

17
The suicidal patient–doctor relationship

Danuta Wasserman

Introduction

The relationship that develops between the patient and the doctor in the course of the suicide risk assessment has a crucial bearing on the quality of the assessment. The process that arises in every interpersonal relationship is known as 'transference'. In transference, the previous perceptions, experiences and unconscious wishes of those involved come to the fore and their usual relationship patterns and conflicts are reactivated. Conflicts and ways of relating to others can be staged in an unconscious or only partially conscious way. In psychiatric terminology, the patient's manner of reacting is known as 'transference' and the doctor's or therapist's response as 'countertransference'.[1]

The suicidal patient's transference

Many suicidal patients complicate all their relationships, including that with the doctor, whom they may see as a saviour or an enemy. The patient may expect love and appreciation but also disparagement. The expectation of receiving help immediately, or that help will never be forthcoming, may also characterize the assessment situation.

A suicidal patient's expectations may be expressed in various ways. Many suicidal patients do not seek help or co-operate well. Some patients may have a negative attitude and show a hostile, silent and rejecting attitude towards the doctor in the assessment situation. Others may be provocative or 'act superior'. These reactions may occur because earlier perceptions of rejection and disapproval and memories of narcissistic injury, of being snubbed or feeling like an outsider have arisen in the patient's mind. Leaving or rejecting others then seems preferable to being left.

Some suicidal patients may be entirely indifferent to whether they live or die. Still others may have exaggerated expectations that the doctor can 'fix everything' and these patients are easily disappointed.[2]

Interaction between the suicidal patient's and doctor's ambivalence

Suicidal patients are highly ambivalent. They swing from wanting to die to wanting to live and between despair and hope. Sometimes, during the short assessment, only the positive side of the ambivalence is manifested and the negative side can be missed altogether. A suicidal person's ambivalence may interact with the ambivalence of the doctor performing the assessment. This is expressed in the doctor's perception of only the patient's strength and not the need for care, or only the patient's weakness, in which case there is a risk of the doctor exerting too much control over the patient. Sometimes, a doctor's ambivalence towards a suicidal patient may result in the doctor misjudging or completely missing a suicide risk, owing to a kind of unconscious consensus arising between the patient, who is reluctant to display his or her vulnerability, and the doctor, who is unwilling to recognize the patient's suicidality.[3,4]

Patients may hide their needs

In a structured and soothing assessment situation, suicidal people may temporarily calm down and cease to show their desperation or to communicate their profound suicidal ideation or suicide plans, however marked they may be. This may be because of a sense of shame or a temporary feeling that all may perhaps be well.

Many suicidal people are reluctant to show their vulnerability and try to manage without the help of others, hiding their feelings of uncertainty and inferiority.[5] Not infrequently, this kind of attitude develops in childhood. As children, these patients were very often obliged to cope on their own without being capable of doing so.

In a desperate situation, despite strong reflections about suicide and an acute need for the help they seek, they may repress their suicidality. Consequently, unless exploratory questions are asked, suicidality is not detected if the doctor is neither inclined nor trained to recognize it.[3,4]

The doctor's countertransference

Doctors are unavoidably influenced by their patients' transference and projections. Like all human beings, doctors have various personality traits, characters and psychological conflicts. They assess suicide risk and the need for admission, nursing and treatment not only according to their professional knowledge but also according to their individual qualities and values, as well as their attitudes to life, death and suicidality.

Many employees in the health-care services choose their occupation out of fear of death, dependence and helplessness. Suicidal patients' self-destructive behaviour runs counter to the instinct of self-preservation, and the desire to cure and alleviate, that are so strongly developed in most health-care staff. Partly as a result of this, doctors may, in a verbal or non-verbal way and both unconsciously and consciously, show disapproval of patients who have attempted suicide or have plans to commit suicide.

Most doctors feel empathy and exhibit interest, when performing assessment of suicide risk and are capable to establish a sound relationship with a suicidal patient. However, there are also doctors who may be extremely frightened and see suicide risk everywhere. They 'persecute' patients in an insensitive way with questions about suicidal ideation and suicide attempts. Instead of winning patients' confidence and motivating them to undergo treatment, they frighten them away.

Other doctors may be indifferent, uncommitted, unobservant and passive in their approach. Yet others may have an exaggerated sense of helplessness and think that there is nothing they can do. Not infrequently, doctors who are of a depressive disposition can adopt such an attitude and even become suicidal themselves. Others may feel questioned in their professional role and conclude that they are bad at their job when their narcissistic feeling is threatened.

Sometimes a doctor may have a strong desire to be rid of the patient, whom they perceive as provocative and frustrating to deal with. In some cases, doctors may even show dismissive and negative attitudes and reject the patient. This kind of attitude may be a manifestation of the doctor's unresolved, underlying aggressive conflicts.[1,6]

Role assigned to the doctor

The role assigned to doctors and therapists by the patient, and the patient's reactions to them, do not only involve repetition of the patient's old conflicts or patterns. These reactions also depend on the current emotional attitude of the doctor who meets them, which may precipitate the patient's transference reaction.

Doctors' own mental conflicts influence their feelings towards a suicidal person and may impede the assessment of suicide risk. Awareness of one's 'blind spots' prevents misinterpretations. Doctors and therapists who have a good knowledge of their own psychological functioning (fostered by training, regular supervision and teamwork) may be able to use their own personality as an asset in the assessment and treatment process and to manage trying emotions experienced by both their patients and themselves.

Difficulties in suicide-risk assessment

Assessing suicide risk is difficult because suicidal people are full of inconsistencies and contradictions.[7] Their thoughts often flit back and forth from one subject, feeling and argument to another.

Suicidal patients' denial of reality and their ambivalence, not only about life and death but also about any form of treatment, may be hard for the assessing doctor to deal with. The same applies to aggressive and manipulative reactions, which are not uncommon in suicidal patients. Being alternately idealized and disparaged, subjected to various provocations and tested to see how much one 'cares' and how much effort one is inclined to make may be very trying.

In assessing suicide risk, it is essential to be aware of suicidal patients' characteristics – their vulnerability, their exaggerated tendency to take offence, their shame and sense of guilt, their marked emotional liability and their tendency to respond with a rejecting attitude as soon as they have the slightest perception that one does not care about them. Doctors need to be trained in showing empathy, giving comfort and reacting in a friendly way, since this greatly assists the implementation of adequate suicide-risk assessment.

Through dialogue with friendly words, one can help suicidal people to verbalize perceptions that they have difficulty in pinning down and turning into words. This is the basis of interpersonal communication and the best way to help in integration of fragmented thoughts and emotions. In suicide-risk assessment, it is also vital to assess what kind of needs have been frustrated, since it is these unsatisfied needs that fuel suicidal ideation and suicide plans.

References

1. Wolk-Wasserman D. Some problems connected with the treatment of suicide attempt patients: transference and countertransference aspects. *Crisis* 1987;**8:** 69–82.

2. Wolk-Wasserman D. The intensive care unit and the suicide attempt patient. *Acta Psychiatr Scand* 1985;**71:**581–595.

3. Wolk-Wasserman D. Contacts of suicidal neurotic and prepsychotic/psychotic patients and their significant others with public care institutions before the suicide attempt. *Acta Psychiatr Scan* 1987;**75:**358–372.

4. Wolk-Wasserman D. Contacts of suicidal alcohol and drug abuse patients and the significant others with public care institutions before their suicide attempt. *Acta Psychiatr Scan* 1987;**76:** 394–405.

5. Henseler H. Narzisstische Krisen. Zur Psychodynamik des Selbstmords. [Narcissistic Crises. On the Psychodynamics of Suicide.]

Hamburg; Rowholt Taschenbuch Verlag; 1974.

6. Maltsberger JT, Buie DH. Countertransference hate in the treatment of suicidal patients. *Arch Gen Psychiatry* 1974;**30:**625–633.

7. Maris R, Berman A, Maltsberger J, Yufit R. Assessment and prediction of suicide. London: Guilford Press; 1992.

18
Psychometric scales in suicide risk assessment

Per Bech, Lis Raabaek Olsen and Anders Niméus

Measurement of suicidal behaviour

Suicidal behaviour can be considered either as a symptom of depressive illness like other depressive symptoms (suicidal thoughts) or as a lack of coping with acute or chronic stress (including poor physical health, social isolation, work problems, family problems and alcohol problems).

Psychometric scales to be used in the daily clinical setting should be simple and brief – the number of items should be 10 or less. The items should obviously have a high degree of content validity; that is, they should cover the relevant domains of the dimension under investigation (e.g. suicide risk). Conventionally, the total score of the items is the sufficient measure (i.e. a higher score means a higher risk of suicide). The reliability of a psychometric scale depends on its administration. Interview or clinician-rated scales should be tested for inter-rater reliability while self-reported questionnaires can be tested for intraindividual reliability by test–retest coefficients.

Psychiatric domains of suicidal behaviour

When reviewing the psychometric scales developed up to 1985, Bürk et al. identified nine domains covered by the selected 15 scales.[1] The most comprehensive scale with the ability to distinguish between previous suicide attempters and non-attempters was developed by Zung – the Zung Index of Potential Suicide.[2] This scale included 19 demographic and 50 clinical variables. However, Petrie and Chamberlain found that only the clinical variables of depression and hopelessness had some predictive validity.[3]

Table 18.1 shows the three brief scales in the meta-analysis of Bürk et al.[1] These scales are brief without losing screening validity. Of these three scales, the Risk Estimator for Suicide covers domains that describe demographic data, evidence of mental disorders, previous suicidal

147

Table 18.1   Comparison of three brief suicide prediction scales. The sensitivity and specificity data in (A) are from Bürk et al.[1] and those in (B) are from Rothberg and Geer-Williams.[8]

Domains		Risk Estimator for Suicide[4]		Risk of Repetition Scale[5]	Post-Attempt Risk Assessment Scale[6,9]
Demographic data		+		+	+
Evidence of mental disorders		+		+	
Previous suicidal behaviour		+		+	+
Social isolation		+		+	+
Poor physical health		+			
Stressors		+			
Number of items		15		6	6
Sufficient score index		Weighted total score		Simple total score	Weighted total score
(A) Screening validity	Sensitivity	Males	0.60–0.80	0.83–0.88	0.81–0.83
		Females	0.32–0.75		
	Specificity	Males	0.52–0.84	0.24–0.44	0.74–0.84
		Females	0.84–0.85		
(B) Screening validity	Sensitivity			0.63–0.73	0.83
	Specificity			0.63–0.78	0.67–0.83

behaviour, social isolation, poor physical health and stressors.[4] The Risk of Repetition Scale[5] covers four domains, while the Post-attempt Risk Assessment Scale[6] covers only three domains. However, these three domains (demographic data, previous suicidal behaviour and social isolation) are also covered by the two other scales. Among these three domains, the Post-attempt Risk Assessment Scale is the one that has the best sensitivity and specificity when used by the clinician as a screening instrument.

The domain of previous suicidal behaviour reflects the fact that previous suicidal behaviour is itself the most valid measurement. It is analogous to depressive illness in which previous episodes of depression are the most powerful predictor of future major depression. Social isolation is also a well-known risk factor of suicide. Among the demographic variables, male sex and alcohol problems are similarly known as risk factors of suicide.

Table 18.2 shows the Risk of Repetition Scale.[5] The scale relies relatively heavily on evidence of mental disorders.

Table 18.3 shows the Post-attempt Risk Assessment Scale.[6] This scale places the highest weight on previous suicidal attempts, followed by social class, sex and social isolation. The inter-rater reliability of the Post-attempt Risk Assessment Scale is acceptable. It has been suggested[6] that the scale should be used together with the first part of the Suicidal Intent Scale developed by Beck et al.[7]

Table 18.2   Risk of Repetition Scale.

Item number	Item	Score
1	Distress felt by other than the subject	(0–1)
2	Problems with alcohol	(0–1)
3	Previous in-patient psychiatric treatment	(0–1)
4	Previous out-patient psychiatric treatment	(0–1)
5	Previous attempted suicide resulting in hospitalization	(0–1)
6	Not living with a relative	(0–1)
	Total score	(0–6)

Scoring: 0, absent; 1, present.
Higher total score, higher risk.
Modified from Buglass and Horton.[5]

Table 18.3   Post-attempt Risk Assessment Scale.

Item number	Item		Weighted score	Score
1	Age	Up to 44 years	0.1	
		45 years or more	5.0	
2	Sex	Male	6.4	
		Female	5.0	
3	Social class	Upper	6.6	
		Lower	5.0	
4	Work status	Employed	2.7	
		Retired	2.4	
		Other	5.0	
5	Living arrangements	Alone	5.8	
		Not alone	5.0	
6	Suicidal communication in the last year	Yes	7.5	
		No	5.0	

Modified after Pallis et al.[6,9]

Classification of suicide attempters

The Suicidal Intent Scale was not included in the meta-analysis by Bürk et al.[1] because the scale is not a suicide risk scale but rather a scale to be used in research studies to classify attempters. The first part of the scale focuses on the objective circumstances related to the suicide attempt. This part has a high inter-rate reliability. The second part covers the patient's personally reported feelings prior to as well as after the attempt.

Suicidal thoughts and impulses

The Scale for Suicide Ideation was developed by Beck et al.[10] to measure the severity of suicidal thoughts. It is an interview-rated scale consisting of 19 items. Each item can be scored from 0 to 2; therefore the theoretical score ranges from 0 to 38. Higher scores signify more suicidal thoughts.

The psychometric description of the current form of the Scale for Suicide Ideation (SSI-C) is shown in Figure 18.1. The inter-rater reliability is adequate and the internal consistency (validity) is high, with a coefficient-alpha of 0.89. This means that some items are redundant.

Its external validity when it is measuring changes in suicidal thoughts over time (responsiveness of the psychometric scale) is also acceptable. Therefore, the SSI-C correlates significantly both with a symptom-rating scale (Beck Depression Inventory) and with the symptom of hopelessness (Beck Hopelessness Scale, Beck et al.[12]).

Factor analysis of the SSI-C has identified three factors as indicative of measurements of suicidal risk: active suicidal thoughts, preparation and passive suicidal thoughts.

In conclusion, the SSI-C measures the intensity of suicidal thoughts analogously to rating scales for the measurement of depressive symptoms. Table 18.4 shows the suicide items in the Hamilton Depression Rat-

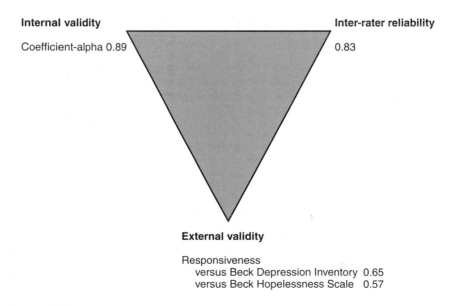

Internal validity

Coefficient-alpha 0.89

Inter-rater reliability

0.83

External validity

Responsiveness
versus Beck Depression Inventory 0.65
versus Beck Hopelessness Scale   0.57

Figure 18.1
Psychometric triangle describing the Scale for Suicide Ideation (SSI-C).

Table 18.4   Suicide items in the Hamilton Depression Rating Scale (HAM-D).

Score	Item
0	No suicidal thoughts
1	The patient feels that life is not worthwhile, but he or she expresses no wish to die
2	The patient wishes to die but has no plans for taking his or her own life
3	It is probable that the patient contemplates committing suicide
4	During the days before the interview the patient has tried to commit suicide or the patient is under special observation because of suicide risk

From Bech et al.[11]

ing Scale (HAM-D). In clinical trials with major depression, a score of 3 or more on this item excludes patients in placebo-controlled studies because of the high risk of suicide.

In 1999 Beck et al. published the Scale for Suicide Ideation with a measure of the suicidal thoughts at the worst point in the patient's life (SSI-W).[13] Compared with SSI-C and the Beck Hopelessness Scale, the SSI-W was superior in predicting suicide.

Quality of life, depressed mood, hopelessness, and distress

Hopelessness

The Beck Hopelessness Scale (BHS) is one of the most frequently used self-reported questionnaires for the prediction of suicide. The scale consists of 20 items, each of which is rated true or false. Thus, the total score has a theoretical range from 0 to 20 and people with a score of 10 or more have a high risk of suicide. However, the false positive rate is extremely high even when using a score of 17 or more.

Figure 18.2 shows a psychometric description of the BHS. The internal consistency (validity) is extremely high, indicating that some items are redundant. To the best of our knowledge the test–retest reliability of the BHS has not been reported. The external (concurrent) validity shows a high correlation with the Beck Depression Inventory (see Figure 18.2). The symptom of hopelessness is included in the items of depressed mood in the HAM-D (Table 18.5). However, hopelessness is a subjective experience, which is measured most appropriately with a questionnaire such as the BHS rather than by the HAM-D. However, even with clinician-rated depression scales, the BHS has a higher positive correlation with hopelessness.

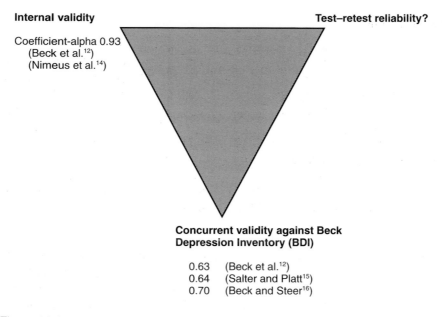

Internal validity

Coefficient-alpha 0.93
(Beck et al.[12])
(Nimeus et al.[14])

Test–retest reliability?

**Concurrent validity against Beck
Depression Inventory (BDI)**

0.63   (Beck et al.[12])
0.64   (Salter and Platt[15])
0.70   (Beck and Steer[16])

Figure 18.2

Psychometric triangle describing the Beck Hopelessness Scale (BHS).

Table 18.5   Depressed mood items in the Hamilton Depression Rating Scale (HAM-D).

Score	Item
0	Neutral mood
1	It is doubtful whether the patient is more despondent or sad than usual (e.g. the patient indicates vaguely that he or she is more depressed than usual)
2	The patient more clearly is concerned by unpleasant experiences, although he or she is still without helplessness or hopelessness
3	The patient shows clear non-verbal signs of depression and/or is at times overpowered by helplessness or hopelessness
4	The patient's remarks on despondency and helplessness or the non-verbal signs dominate the interview and the patient cannot be distracted from them

From Bech et al.[11]

Quality of life

Quality of life is defined as a subjective, psychological dimension.[17] Meta-analysis of various quality-of-life questionnaires has shown that the general factor or dimension is positive versus negative psychological well-being, as in the Psychological General Well-Being Scale (PGWB).[18]

The BHS is constructed, as is the PGWB, with items that cover both positive and negative coping. Nine of the BHS items measure positive coping (keyed 'false'). The other 11 BHS items measure negative coping or well-being (keyed 'true') (e.g. 'My future seems dark').

Within quality-of-life research, questionnaires seem to measure only positive well-being. The World Health Organization Well-Being Scale constructed by Bech covers five of the 22 items in the PGWB.

Distress

Distress can be defined as negative psychological well-being. The Hopkins Symptom Checklist (SCL-90) is a measure of distress that consists of several psychological subscales. In a group of psychiatric patients who had previously attempted suicide, SCL-90 showed its ability to distinguish between reattempters and non-reattempters.

Table 18.6 shows a checklist in which the acronym refers to the ten domains identified in Tables 18.1—18.5. This is the SAD PERSONS scale developed by Patterson et al.[19] Hopelessness is included in the item of depressed mood. Suicidal thoughts and impulses are included in the item of organized plan for suicide. The SAD PERSONS scale has not been evaluated psychometrically. However, on the basis of the total

Table 18.6   The SAD PERSONS Scale for assessing the risk of suicide.

Acronym and domain (if present, score 1)	Score
Sex (male)	(0–1)
Age (younger than 20 years or older than 45 years)	(0–1)
Depressed mood	(0–1)
Previous suicide attempt	(0–1)
Ethanol abuse	(0–1)
Rational thinking loss (e.g. organic brain syndrome, affective disorders, schizophrenia)	(0–1)
Social support lacking	(0–1)
Organized plan for suicide	(0–1)
No spouse or not living with a relation	(0–1)
Sickness, poor physical health	(0–1)
Total score	(0–10)

When assessing a person in the emergency room, the total score guidelines are: 0–2, send home with follow-up; 3–4, close follow-up; 5–6, strongly consider hospitalization; 7–10, hospitalization.
From Patterson et al.[19] modified to cover Tables 18.1–18.5.

score, guidelines for clinical action are used (see Table 18.6). A modified version has obtained a sensitivity of 94% and a specificity of 74% when identifying the need of hospitalization.

Clinical use of psychometric scales

This overview has analysed the psychometric domains of suicidal behaviour from a pragmatic, clinical point of view. Most of the scales that have been mentioned are brief, interview-rated instruments that cover such domains as previous attempts, demographic data, social isolation and current psychopathology (suicidal thoughts and depressed mood) (see Table 18.6). These domains are all within the body of evidence concerning risk factors for suicide. The total scores of the various scales have a high sensitivity for prediction but their specificity is lower.

The only self-rating questionnaire that has been frequently used is the BHS. It has a high applicability across the various populations in which it has been used. The scale can be compared to psychological well-being scales by measuring a dimension of positive versus negative satisfaction, coping or well-being. The BHS is an example of a generic quality-of-life questionnaire that measures the dimension of positive versus negative well-being or coping across individuals in different settings.

Kehoe and Gutheil[20] have criticized the generic scales that assess suicidal risk because of their neglect of religious dimension, which is a unique individual domain that is important in the therapy of suicidal persons. Of the scales reviewed here, only the Zung Index of Potential Suicide includes items of religion.

Among the most fruitful psychometric scales to measure individual quality of life is the Repertory Grid Technique developed by Kelly.[21] The idiographic approach in the Repertory Grid Technique is the free construct, which supplements the fixed constructs or domains covered by the generic scales.

Table 18.7 shows the clinical issues that can be extracted from the generic suicide scale analysed in this review. The suicidal thought or ideation is listed as the element by which the fixed and free constructs are measured on Visual Analogue Scales. The fixed constructs are very similar to those used in quality-of-life scales, while religion is used as an example of a free construct.

Clinician and self-reported scales

This overview has identified the domains or constructs covered by brief rating scales developed for the measurement of suicidal risk. The clinician-rated scales cover such domains as previous attempts, demo-

Table 18.7   Repertory grid.

Elements (suicidal thoughts)	Fixed constructs						Free constructs
	Physical health	Hopelessness	Affective mood	Social isolation	Economic situation	Self-awareness	Religion
At its worst point in your life	0–100	0–100	0–100	0–100	0–100	0–100	0–100
Today	0–100	0–100	0–100	0–100	0–100	0–100	0–100
In a period without suicidal thoughts	0–100	0–100	0–100	0–100	0–100	0–100	0–100

Each grid is measured by the subject on a Visual Analogue Scale from 0, worst thinkable to 100, best thinkable.

graphic data, social isolation and current psychopathology. The self-reported scales concentrate on hopelessness, which is an individual, psychological experience.

The Repertory Grid Technique is a psychometric method of measuring the individual or idiographic approach in analysing what is of importance for the subject under evaluation, although this might not be considered important by other people such as the patient's relatives or the doctor. The religious dimension is an example of the idiographic approach. Suicidal thought or ideation is the quantifier of the domains, fixed as well as free.

References

1. Bürk F, Kurz A, Möller HJ. Suicide risk scales: do they help to predict suicidal behaviour? *Eur Arch Psychiatr Neurol Sci* 1985;**235:** 153–157.

2. Zung WWK. Index of Potential Suicide (IPS). In: Beck AT, Resnik HLP, Lettieri D (eds). The prediction of suicide. Maryland: Charles Press; 1974:221–249.

3. Petrie K, Chamberlain K. The predictive validity of the Zung Index of Potential Suicide. *J Pers Assess* 1985;**49:**100–102.

4. Motto JA, Heilbron DC. Development and validation of scales for estimation of suicidal risk. In: Schneidman E (ed). Suicidology, contemporary developments. New York: Grune and Stratton; 1976:169–199.

5. Buglass D, Horton J. A scale for predicting subsequent suicidal behaviour. *Br J Psychiatry* 1974;**124:**573–578.

6. Pallis DJ, Gibbons JS, Pierce DW. Estimating suicide risk among attempted suicides. II. Efficiency of predictive scales after the attempt. *Br J Psychiatry* 1984; **144:**139–148.

7. Beck AT, Schnyler D, Herman J. Development of suicidal intent scales. In: Beck AT, Resnik HLP, Lettieri DJ (eds). The prediction of

suicide. Maryland: Charles Press; 1974a:45–56.

8. Rothberg JM, Geer-Williams C. A comparison and review of suicide prediction scales. In: Marris RW, Berman AL, Maltsberger JT, Yufit RI (eds). Assessment and prediction of suicide. New York: Guildford Press; 1992:202–217.

9. Pallis DJ, Barraclough MB, Levey AB et al. Estimating suicide risk among attempted suicides: 1. The development of new clinical scales. *Br J Psychiatry* 1982;**141:** 37–44

10. Beck AT, Kovacs M, Weissmann A. Assessment of suicidal intention: the Scale for Suicide Ideation. *J Consult Clin Psychology* 1979;**46:**343–352.

11. Bech P, Kastrup M, Rafaelsen OJ. Mini-compendium of rating scales for states of anxiety, depression, mania, schizophrenia with corresponding DSM-III syndromes. *Acta Psychiatr Scand* 1986; **73(Suppl 326):**7–37.

12. Beck AT, Weisman A, Lester D, Trexler L. The measurement of pessimism. The Hopelessness Scale. *J Consult Clin Psychol* 1974b;**41:**861–865.

13. Beck AT, Brown GK, Steer RA, et al. Suicide ideation at its worst point: a predictor of eventual

suicide in psychiatric outpatients. *Suicide Life Threat Behav* 1999;**29:**1–9.

14. Nimeus A, Träskman-Bendz L, Alsen M. Hopelessness and suicidal behavior. J Affect Disord 1997;**42:**137–144.

15. Salter D, Platt S. Suicidal intent, hopelessness and depression in a parasuicidal population: the influence of social desirability and elapsed time. *Br J Clin Psychol* 1990;**29:**361–371.

16. Beck AT, Steer RA. Manual for the Beck Hopelessness Scale. San Antonio TACKSAM: Psychological Corporation; 1993.

17. Bech P. Quality of life in the psychiatric patient. London: Mosby-Wolfe; 1998.

18. Bech P. Rating scales for psychopathology, health status, and quality of life. A compendium with correspondence to DSM-III-R and the WHO. Berlin: Springer; 1993.

19. Patterson WM, Dohn HH, Bird J, Patterson GA. Evaluation of suicide patients: the SAD PERSONS scale. *Psychosomatics* 1983;**24:** 343–352.

20. Kehoe NC, Gutheil TG. Neglect of religious issues in scale-based assessment of suicidal patients. Hosp Community Psychiatry 1994;**45:**366–369.

21. Kelly GA. The psychology of personal constructs. Vol 1: A theory of personality. Vol 2: Clinical diagnosis and psychotherapy. New York: Norton; 1955 and London: Routledge; 1991.

Section V
Treatment

19

Psychological treatment of suicidal patients

Paul M Salkovskis

Introduction

Almost all patients who have made a suicide attempt or who are explicitly identified as seriously contemplating suicide elicit efforts from those around them that are intended to provide psychological help or to dissuade them from any further suicidal actions. Such interventions range from overt hostility through to obvious care and sympathy, from practical help with problems through to detention or even imprisonment. The intention can be to help or to punish. It is clear that people who are actively suicidal seldom leave those around them unmoved. Usually, both professionals and non-professionals experience a sense of dismay, failure and helplessness.

Unfortunately, the psychological value of different ways of responding is not well understood. As a result, psychological approaches to suicide prevention vary widely from telephone helplines through to strategies designed to make psychiatric services more accessible by the provision of priority cards. At its most intense, service provision involves structured in-patient or out-patient psychotherapy services that are supposedly tailored to the needs of the suicidal patients but that are more often based on clinical folklore and supposition. Only two focused psychotherapeutic approaches have so far been found to be helpful in controlled trials with people at risk of attempting suicide. These two approaches are:

- cognitive–behavioural therapy (CBT), particularly problem solving approaches; and
- dialectical behaviour therapy (DBT).

The fact that there is considerable overlap between these two effective approaches is probably not a coincidence. Evidence for the effectiveness of other forms of psychotherapy is sparse, although research on factors associated with suicide attempts suggests that there may be a case for further investigation of approaches such as interpersonal psychotherapy. There are theoretical and clinical reasons why there has

161

been so little progress in the effective treatment of those who have attempted suicide or who are at risk of further attempts, despite considerable effort having been made over many years. It is now reasonable to hope that an understanding of these factors will lead to the development and delivery of better psychological treatments.

Effective treatment for people who attempt suicide: understanding and helping

The development of behavioural therapies and CBT over the past decade has radically changed the outlook throughout the field of psychotherapy. The prospect of brief, specifically focused, effective and efficient treatment has now become a reality.[1] This progress has been achieved through the use of a systematic strategy that can be characterized as being based on 'clinical science'. Although this approach need not necessarily be unique to CBT, no other school of psychotherapy currently applies it.

The clinical science approach is underpinned by an understanding of the specific phenomenology of clinical problems, which is not only linked to well-defined theory of the specific problem but is also backed by experimental studies of psychopathology and studies of treatment outcome. A further factor is the basis of cognitive–behavioural approaches in assumptions that have substantially diverged from (and sometimes even contradict) those implicit in more traditional psychotherapies. In particular, it is assumed that treatment will be effective only if it deals with the factors that maintain the person's problems. Although attention to aetiological factors may be useful at times, it is seldom, if ever, found to be essential in cognitive-behavioural therapies. Cognitive–behavioural approaches also assume that there is very considerable specificity in the factors involved in the maintenance of particular disorders, and that an understanding of such specificity is crucial to guiding the therapist, who works collaboratively with the patient to devise and implement an individualized programme of treatment. Thus, the treatment of a depressed patient is guided by a specific understanding of mechanisms that are involved in the maintenance of the symptoms of depression, and it has a quite different focus and emphasis from that of the treatment of a patient suffering from panic attacks, which would in turn also differ from a person suffering from bulimia nervosa, and so on. This requirement for specific focus is quite different from the targets usually defined in more generic types of psychotherapy, sharing only what CBT would regard as basic psychotherapeutic skills (such as the ability to react in an empathic way).

Forming a good therapeutic relationship and alliance enable therapy and are necessary for it to be conducted properly, but they are not sufficient, do not form the primary focus of it and are not defined as the main mechanism of change. Indeed, recent research suggests that a good therapeutic alliance may be a consequence rather than a cause of clinical effectiveness. These considerations also have important implications for the training of psychotherapists.

Psychological factors maintaining suicidal ideation

The development of effective and specific treatments of people who attempt suicide (or who might go on to kill themselves) therefore may require a clear understanding of the mechanisms characteristic of people who persistently manifest suicidal ideation and behaviour.[2] Ways of helping these people flow directly from this understanding. Two prominent cognitive mechanisms have so far been identified in patients who have made suicide attempts. The first of these mechanisms involves deficits in problem-solving skills, particularly interpersonal problem solving. Secondly, there is evidence of a bias towards retrieval of over-general (as opposed to specific) memories. In addition, there is evidence for a third factor, which is the association between feelings of hopelessness and actual suicide. It follows that treatments that modify such factors should be effective in helping people who are troubled by suicidal ideation and effective in reducing both the rate of repeat attempts and the rate of actual suicide. Consideration of these three psychological maintaining factors also suggests that they are not fully independent, an observation confirmed by a number of research studies. The identification of links between the key maintaining factors may hold the key to the development of focused and integrated psychological treatment.

Problem-solving deficits in suicidal persons

Although there is relatively strong evidence that problem-solving deficits may have a specific association with attempted suicide,[3,4] problem solving is characterized by a complex and interacting set of processes (such as problem definition, generating solutions and implementing the chosen solution). Unfortunately, it is not clear which processes or sub-processes are impaired. By contrast, problems with over-general memories are easier to define, but evidence for the specificity of such deficits is not good; deficits that are found may be related to increased levels of depression and distress in the target group rather than to suicidality *per se*.

An appealing possibility links problem-solving deficits and over-general memory retrieval. The process of problem solving involves the retrieval of several different types of memory, including the particular problem or problems to be solved, strategies that have previously been successful, the practical steps required for the effective deployment of such strategies, and the pre-existing resources and assets which could be deployed in problem solving. Problem-solving therapies stress the importance of specificity in successful problem. It may be that problem-solving deficits arise from the tendency towards over-general memory, or, more likely, that the two factors interact. It also seems reasonable to speculate that perceived problem-solving deficits (whether real or not) contribute to hopelessness.[5] Fortunately, effective treatment need not await resolution of these issues, since problem-solving training with a cognitive–behavioural emphasis is likely to deal not only with problem-solving deficits *per se*, but also with impairments in the ability to generate specific (as opposed to over-general) memories.

Problem solving in CBT

There is considerable consensus about the most effective ways of helping patients to learn focused problem-solving strategies.[6] These are appropriately based on current psychological knowledge of how 'normal' problem solving is conducted. As with other forms of CBT, the aim of problem-solving treatment is to empower the person so that whatever is learnt in the process of psychological therapy can be flexibly applied to later and other situations. The therapist seeks to motivate the person's engagement in problem-solving attempts by identifying the way in which the person's past and current distress has arisen from identifiable and potentially soluble problems that interfere with the ability to realize important personal and interpersonal goals. This may be in terms of a crisis, in which the blockage is acutely imposed (as with the occurrence of adverse life events) or more chronic problems, perhaps linked to generally poor or even counterproductive coping strategies. This latter group includes those people who are defined as suffering from 'personality disorders' and skills deficits.

Once the link between problem-solving deficits and distress is made, the person is encouraged to recognize his or her existing strengths and resources, and to consider how these might be advantageously deployed. An explicit problem-solving strategy is then identified. Although this strategy is usually modified to fit with the particular person being helped, it generally follows a format that includes:

- making a problem list;
- prioritizing problems to be dealt with, not only on the basis of importance and impact but also on the basis of likely short-term effectiveness;
- deciding on a range of possible solutions, usually involving an element of unconstrained 'brainstorming', in which the person is encouraged to consider freely any possible solution;

- selecting a particular solution, often by systematically reviewing the pros and cons of the most likely solutions available;
- breaking down the implementation of the chosen solution into smaller, more manageable steps;
- anticipating and identifying obstacles to each step (including not only practical difficulties, but also cognitive and emotional difficulties); and
- systematically reviewing progress between steps before deciding whether to move on to the next step.

During the problem-solving process, the therapist helps the patient to re-frame any difficulties as learning opportunities and to try out new ways of overcoming obstacles to problem solving. In this way, the process becomes iterative, with the desired end-result being that the patient has learned not only how to solve specific problems, but has also learned to solve problems that occur during the problem-solving process. The person therefore learns not only how to solve the particular problem that has been focused on in treatment, but also how to apply a more systematic problem-solving strategy. Throughout this process, the importance of specificity in thinking about solutions and their implementation is emphasized. In this way, both problem-solving deficits and deficits in specificity of recall may be corrected by treatment. It also seems likely that problem solving has the effect of reducing hopelessness in people who have previously been unable to see any way out of what had seemed to be insoluble situations.

Effectiveness of CBT

In a small clinical study of people who had not only recently made a suicide attempt but who were also identified as being at high risk of making repeated suicide attempts, a very brief CBT-based problem-solving treatment was shown by Salkovskis et al.[7] in 1990 to be more effective than 'treatment as usual'. Significantly more reductions were obtained not only in the rate of repetition of suicide attempt, but also in levels of depression and hopelessness and an individualized measure of personally defined problems. In addition, there was evidence that there was also a significant reduction in those problems that were not targeted during therapy, suggesting that there was some generalization of problem-solving skills used in the course of therapy. Interestingly, a similarly designed and implemented study, conducted by Atha et al.[8] in 1992 from the same research group, demonstrated that problem-solving treatment was completely ineffective for patients attending an emergency medical facility for reasons other than suicide attempts. These results are consistent with the notion of therapy specificity, described above. In patients who are at risk of suicide, this approach has the considerable merits of being very brief (between five and 10 sessions) and of having surprisingly broad impact, not only in terms of obtaining problem solutions and reducing suicide attempts, but also in terms of reduced levels of psychopathology, including both depression and hopelessness. This latter finding goes some way towards dealing with concerns about the relative narrowness of the focus of this approach to therapy. When persistent symptoms of major depression is an issue in patients who attempt suicide, it may be important to consider broadening the treatment approach to incorporate 'standard cognitive therapy' focused on dealing with depression itself.

Dialectal behaviour therapy

Our current understanding of the mechanisms involved in suicidal ideation and behaviour is complicated by the issue of diagnosis, not only by depression but also by 'personality disorder', which is sometimes (but definitely not always) associated with a tendency towards suicidal behaviour. DBT was introduced by Linehan[9] in 1993 and is designed to help patients suffering from 'borderline personality disorder' who are chronically parasuicidal. This approach shares many features and procedures of cognitive–behavioural problem solving but is a much more broadly based and complex therapy package. Linehan manages to deal with many of the problems associated with the use of the concept of 'personality disorder'. She identifies emotional dysregulation as a key factor that arises from biologically vulnerable patients being exposed at an early age to invalidating environments. The resulting affective instability then interacts with instability in behavioural, interpersonal and cognitive domains to produce the pattern of reactions that are characteristic of such patients, including parasuicidal behaviour. Thus, borderline personality disorder is used as an umbrella term to cover a wide range of relatively enduring problems in the way in which some people seek to cope with their interpersonal and emotional difficulties.

Core skills

Unlike many other approaches to personality disorder, DBT actively seeks to avoid 'blaming the victim'. Treatment focuses on validation and empowerment, consistent with the philosophy of cognitive–behavioural approaches to 'axis 1' disorders. In DBT, the therapist aims to help the patient to modulate his or her emotional reactions, to reduce the associated extreme behaviours and to accept his or her own reactions. Problem solving is a core skills training strategy, supplemented by a range of ancillary treatments, supportive group sessions and telephone consultations. There is a considerably greater emphasis on working on and with the therapeutic relationship (more in the style of cognitive than psychodynamic psychotherapy). Other core skills taught in DBT include mindfulness training, interpersonal effectiveness skills and techniques designed to deal with psychological distress (including well-validated cognitive and behavioural techniques designed to deal with depression, anxiety and post-traumatic stress). Mindfulness training, which involves a series of adapted meditation techniques, has been shown to be separately effective in the management of depression in chronically depressed patients. These techniques are applied in an integrated and formulation-driven way, adapted for use with this particular group of patients in ways that take their particular sensitivities into account.

Effectiveness of DBT

There is good evidence that DBT reduces suicide attempts and service utilization relative to the usual treatment. However, it has a number of disadvantages, including the complexity of the package and the fact that it requires a very considerable input of therapist time (several sessions each week) over a period of up to 1 year. Improvements in terms of measures of psychopathology (such as depression) have been relatively disappointing. Clearly, there is an urgent need for a comparison with the very brief types of problem solving described above, since these have been found to be effective in reducing both suicide attempts and psychopathology, albeit in a somewhat different (and possibly less difficult) patient group.

Interpersonal therapy: a promising prospect

Consideration of the psychopathology of people who attempt suicide (as described above) suggests that interpersonal psychotherapy might also be effective in the treatment of such patients. This expectation arises from two observations:

- interpersonal psychotherapy has been found to be effective in the treatment of depression; and
- interpersonal psychotherapy has a clear emphasis on helping the patient to deal with current interpersonal problems and role transitions in ways that are likely to result in a greater specific focus.

The focus of therapy is on the link between the onset of depressive symptoms and the current interpersonal problems. The emphasis of change strategies is on the person's immediate personal context, his or her reaction to life events and current social dysfunction and how these factors relate to symptom formation. No attempt is made to deal with more enduring aspects of personality. Having established links between interpersonal functioning and depressive symptoms, specific intervention strategies are used according to a detailed manual developed by Klerman and Weissman.[10] Three examples are the way in which unresolved grief is tackled by facilitated mourning, the way in which the patient is guided in the use of interpersonal problem-solving strategies to deal with 'role disputes' in which there is perceived conflict with a significant other, and the way in which 'role transitions' can be focused on as a means of helping the person deal with major life changes. Skills training is a major part of the later stages of interpersonal psychotherapy, and treatment is almost entirely problem focused, with the emphasis firmly in the 'here and now'.

Thus, the specific problem-solving focus of interpersonal psychotherapy makes it attractive as a potential treatment for people who make suicide attempts. However, as yet there have been no published results of its specific effectiveness in this group. Nevertheless, from efficacy documented in terms of dealing with patients who are depressed and in whom life events and interpersonal problems are a major feature, it would be reasonable to infer that this approach may be helpful, possibly as part of a broader integrated package.

The characteristics of effective therapy

How to evaluate

There has been an unfortunate tendency to aggregate psychological treatments for suicide attempters both in terms of the procedures used and the populations evaluated. A recent systematic review by Hawton et al.[11] used a meta-analysis in which a small number of heterogeneous studies were combined in a potentially misleading way. Unfortunately such analyses which are well suited to the systematic evaluation of treatments in which many trials have been conducted with well standardized interventions given to large and homogeneous samples (e.g. in antibiotic treatment of infections) offer a spurious sense of precision which may have the effect of preventing rather than facilitating further developments of promising new treatments. Future research and reviews of research on psychological treatment need to be clear not only about the outcome measures used (which would most appropriately include a range of clinical outcomes, such as hopelessness and suicidal ideation, in addition to the rate of repeat suicide attempts), but also in terms of the populations under investigation and the interventions used. Although efforts to prevent suicide and suicide attempts are probably as old as human life, empirically guided and evaluated treatments are a very recent and sparse development, making techniques such as meta-analysis at best inappropriate for the foreseeable future. At worst, quantitative reviews may be actively misleading in terms of conclusions about the quantitative merits of different treatment approaches relative to each other.

As one would expect given the dearth of outcome research, there is a long list of psychotherapies which have yet to be shown to be effective, or in which there is evidence that they are ineffective in helping people who make suicide attempts. The same problems apply to consideration of the effectiveness of psychotherapeutic approaches to reducing the psychological problems known to be associated with parasuicide in patients at risk of making suicide attempts. These psychological problems include depression, hopelessness, interpersonal problems and persistent emotional reactions to adverse life events.

Criteria of successful psychological treatment

It seems clear at this stage that an active psychological treatment needs to meet the following criteria if it is to have any chance of being successful in reducing the repetition rate of attempted suicide and diminishing the number of successful suicides:

- it must help the patient to feel understood (including, but not confined to, the use of 'non-specific' therapy factors, such as empathy, genuineness and non-possessive warmth, and also including aspects of patient empowerment);
- the main focus of therapeutic efforts should be on factors understood (through empirically grounded theory) to be generally involved in the experience and maintenance of intense and persistent distress in particular patient groups (including, but not confined to, those that meet criteria for particular diagnoses);
- therapy should be adapted to target the particular specific and idiosyncratic manifestations of the generally identified maintaining factors (i.e. the way in which the general maintaining factors affect the particular patient who the therapist is seeking to help); and
- therapy should have been demonstrated to be more effective than a waiting list or treatment as usual.

Currently, only CBT with a problem-solving emphasis and DBT meet all of these criteria. Both standard cognitive therapy for depression and interpersonal therapy currently meet the first three criteria. Given the established effectiveness of both problem cognitive-behavioural solving and the more complex package involved in DBT, the obvious next step in outcome research is a study comparing the much briefer problem-solving approach with DBT, with an additional treatment as usual cell.

Elements that work in psychotherapy of suicidal patients

Interestingly, examination of the details of all four approaches suggests common elements in terms of:

- focus on the 'here and now';
- attention to negative emotions as a guide to the appropriate focus of therapy;
- a major element of both problem-solving and skills training being included in the treatment package; and
- the emphasis being on engaging the person in an empathic, active and collaborative therapeutic relationship in order to empower him or her to make changes to the current situation.

Combination of psychotherapy and medicines

Clinically, the combination of pharmacotherapy and psychotherapy is often used, although one must be aware that pharmacotherapy can increase short-term risk of repetition, because it directly offers the means of suicide attempts by overdose. Offering medication as an acceptable way of resolving the person's distress may also have the effect of decreasing the threshold of acceptability for using medication to persons without psychiatric diagnosis as a more drastic way of resolving their difficulties. There is an urgent need for research into these factors; a better understanding of them might lead to the development of better ways of delivering pharmacotherapy, and may suggest effective ways of combining it with psychotherapy. Although there is some evidence that combining CBT and pharmacotherapy may be helpful in the treatment of depression, recent research on anxiety suggests that the combination may be less effective than CBT alone. There is therefore an urgent need for well conducted research into the factors involved and treatment outcomes; it is astonishing that this has not yet taken place. In the meantime, there is one recent study suggesting that an SSRI (paroxetine) might reduce repetition rates in high risk patients (see Chapter 24). The low toxicity of SSRIs makes them the obvious candidate for combination therapy, at least until the impact of adding medication to psychological treatment is better understood.

Conclusion

There is no need to be hopeless about the treatment of attempted suicide. This chapter began with a discussion of the way in which identification of key maintaining mechanisms has resulted in the rapid evolution of effective and efficient psychotherapeutic approaches to problems such as anxiety disorders. A similar approach has begun to evolve as a major part of efforts to improve the effectiveness of treatment for those who attempt suicide or are at risk of such an attempt, and there is now good evidence for the importance of helping patients to deal with problem-solving deficits and the tendency to retrieve over-general memories. Other important factors that may be related to the understanding (and therefore treatment) of attempted suicide include:

* hopelessness;
* depression; and
* manifestations of 'personality disorder', particularly borderline personality disorder.

Further research is needed to clarify the links between these factors, and how to reduce both suicide attempts and suicide.

The move away from an exclusive emphasis on diagnostic categories is a particularly welcome trend in this field; even with the troubled and troublesome concept of 'personality disorder' there is hope for the empirical identification of psychological mechanisms as shown by Linehan[9] and Williams.[12] There are good reasons to be optimistic about the prospects for engaging, treating and empowering people in whom hopelessness has previously made suicide seem like one of the few options available to them for dealing with their situation.

References

1. Salkovskis PM. Frontiers of cognitive therapy. New York: Guildford Press; 1996.

2. Beck AT, Brown GK, Steer RA, et al. Suicide ideation at its worst point: a predictor of eventual suicide in psychiatric outpatients. *Suicide Life Threat Behav* 1999;**29:**1–9.

3. Pollock LR, Williams JM. Problem solving and suicidal behavior. *Suicide Life Threat Behav* 1998; **28:**375–387.

4. Schotte DE, Clum GA. Problem solving skills in suicidal psychiatric patients. *J Consult Clin Psychol* 1987;**55:**49–54.

5. Cannon B, Mulroy R, Otto MW, et al Dysfunctional attitudes and poor problem solving skills pre-

dict hopelessness in major depression. *J Affect Disord* 1999; **55:**45–49.

6. Hawton KA, Kirk J. Problem solving. In: Hawton KA, Kirk J, Clark DM (eds). Cognitive behaviour therapy for psychiatric problems: a practical guide. Oxford: Oxford University Press; 1989:406–426.

7. Salkovskis PM, Atha C, Storer D. Cognitive–behavioural problem solving in the treatment of patients who repeatedly attempt suicide. A controlled trial. *Br J Psychiatry* 1990;**157:**871–876.

8. Atha C, Salkovskis PM, Storer D. Cognitive-behavioural problem solving in the treatment of patients attending a medical

emergency department: a controlled trial. *J Psychosom Res* 1992;**36:**299–307.

9. Linehan MM. Cognitive–behavioural treatment of borderline personality disorder. New York: Guilford Press; 1993.

10. Klerman GL, Weissman MM. Interpersonal psychotherapy of depression. New York: Basic Books; 1989.

11. Hawton KA, Arensman E,

Townsend E, et al. Deliberate self harm: systematic review of efficacy of psychosocial and pharmacological treatments in preventing repetition. *BMJ* 1998; **317:**441–447.

12. Williams JMG. Personality disorder and the will: a cognitive neuropsychological approach to schizotypal personality. In: Salkovskis PM (ed). Trends in cognitive and behavioural therapies. Chichester: John Wiley; 1996:63–76.

20
Pharmacological treatment of underlying psychiatric disorders in suicidal patients

Hans-Jürgen Möller

Introduction

Besides counselling and other psychotherapeutic approaches (see Chapter 19), psychopharmacological treatment is necessary for many suicidal patients. Pharmacological and somatic interventions (e.g. electroconvulsive therapy) in people at risk of committing suicide are usually aimed either at actual prevention of suicide by mostly sedative–anxiolytic procedures or at specific treatment of a psychic or somatic disorder that may be the underlying cause. However, to date there is no specific somatic treatment of suicidality. Although 5-hydroxyindoleacetic acid levels in cerebrospinal fluid have repeatedly been found to be lower in suicidal patients and patients who have attempted suicide than in controls, the resulting consequences for treatment have not yet been sufficiently investigated. Administration of serotonergic substances in the treatment of suicidality is based on hypotheses regarding the role of serotonin. However, a clear empirical validation of this approach is lacking.[1]

Suicidality and suicidal behaviour mostly occur in one of the following constellations:

- as acute suicidality after psychosocial stress conditions; or
- as acute or chronic suicidality as a symptom or result of a relevant psychiatric disorder.

This chapter describes psychopharmacological approaches in these two conditions.

Abnormal reactions to psychosocial stressors

When suicidality results from abnormal reactions to psychosocial stressors, psychopharmacological interventions are mainly aimed at sedation, anxiolysis, sleep induction or suppression of vegetative symptoms. Benzodiazepines (or in cases of predominant sleep disturbances the modern non-benzodiazepine hypnotics) are in general the treatment of first choice. The selection of the specific compound and of the dose varies according to the individual case. The aim should be to induce not only sedation but also affective–emotional distancing. Some doctors tend to be very restrictive in prescribing benzodiazepines, even in these conditions, because they are afraid of the risk of dependency, which is in fact extremely low. They prefer to use sedating antidepressants, such as doxepine, or low doses of sedating neuroleptics as surrogates. However, given the extraordinary good tolerability of benzodiazepines and the high compliance of patients with these drugs, the risk–benefit assessment should favour the benzodiazepines in these special conditions, especially given the fact that, in general, only short-term medication is needed. An inadequate psychopharmacological regime could induce a high risk of continuation of suicidality, and therefore undertreatment with benzodiazepines, which seems to become a general problem in patients with a need for benzodiazepine treatment,[2] should be avoided. The non-psychopharmacological treatment approach, sometimes suggested on the basis of psychodynamic theories, is not sufficient if there is a clear syndrome-related indication for psychopharmacological treatment (e.g. emotional instability, severe anxiety, depressive mood or other psychiatric illness). In cases of longer-lasting depressive reactions, antidepressants as well as benzodiazepines should be considered. Modern antidepressants with better tolerability than the tricyclic antidepressants should preferably be chosen.

Neuroses and personality disorders

The International Classification of Diseases, 10th revision (ICD-10) avoids the term 'neurosis' and prefers, in its more descriptive approach, terms such as 'generalized anxiety disorder' and 'dysthymia'. However, the term 'neurosis' is still in common clinical use.

In addition to psychotherapeutic procedures, antidepressants are also very often indicated in so-called neurotic disorders, depending on the type and severity of the symptoms. Examples include dysthymia (for which tricyclic antidepressants of the amitriptyline type, monoamine oxidase (MAO) inhibitors or selective serotonin reuptake inhibitors (SSRIs) are used, for example), anxiety disorders (for which imipramine and SSRIs are used, for example) and obsessive compulsive disorders (for which clomipramine and SSRIs are used, for example). However, if suicidality occurs during such disorders, monotherapy is often not sufficient to overcome the critical situation as quickly as possible. Short-term administration of benzodiazepines or other sedatives, neuroleptics along with antidepressants may also be necessary, with the same aims and approach as described above. However, in the case of longer-term administration, it is necessary to be aware of the risk of abuse with the benzodiazepines and of tardive dyskinesia with the neuroleptics.

Personality disorders are frequently associated with chronic, repetitive suicidality. At special risk are histrionic and borderline patients. In general, the efficacy of psychopharmacological treatment of personality disorders is not well established.[3] In borderline cases especially, the occasional risk of paradoxical reactions to benzodiazepines or tricyclic antidepressants should be taken into consideration.[4] In most cases, only treatment of the acute critical condition seems indicated. Benzodiazepines, antidepressants with a sedative–anxiolytic profile or low-potency neuroleptics in small dosages can be administered in this indication as a short-term intervention. It should be taken into account that these suggestions are based on clinical experience but not on clinical trials. Long-term treatment with benzodiazepines should normally be avoided because of the risk of abuse.

There are only very few studies that have investigated whether a medium-term psychopharmacological approach might be useful in the prevention of further suicide attempts in patients with a history of repeated suicide attempts. The studies that have been performed have mostly involved comorbidity with personality disorders of the impulsive, histrionic and borderline type.[5]

Unipolar and bipolar depression

Being tired of life or longing for death are symptoms that occur almost regularly in depression, especially in moderate or severe cases. Furthermore, a large number of patients think about suicidal acts, perform a suicide attempt or even die from suicide. When selecting an antidepressant for suicidal depressive patients, compounds with a sedative profile (e.g. amitriptyline, doxepine, mianserine, remerone) should be favoured; drugs that increase drive, such as MAO inhibitors or desipramine, may increase the risk of suicide.[6] Another aspect of drug selection is that the antidepressant should be safe in overdose, which is proven for drugs such as the SSRIs, mianserine and remerone. If a tricyclic antidepressant is chosen, the smallest package should be prescribed to avoid the risk of lethal intoxication in case of suicidal overdose. Most tricyclic antidepressants have a high risk of fatal outcome if dosages of 1000 mg or more are taken. SSRIs are nowadays seen as first line treatment of depression, particularly under out-patient conditions, especially with respect to tolerability and compliance.[7] It should be remembered that SSRIs have no sedative potential and in some cases even cause agitation. The degree of sedation achieved even by a sedative antidepressant in highly excited suicidal depressive patients is sometimes insufficient, and it may be necessary to coprescribe a benzodiazepine or a sedative neuroleptic.[6] The dose depends on the patient's excitable condition and his or her individual reaction, and it should be chosen so that the inner restlessness and agitation wear off as completely as possible and significant sedation and promotion of nocturnal sleep are achieved. Since the benzodiazepines seem unfavourable in patients with a history of addiction, a sedative neuroleptic (e.g. 50–200 mg thioridazine or 25–100 mg levomepromazine) may be chosen. In the case of delusional depression, highly potent neuroleptics (e.g. 5–10 mg haloperidol per os or parenterally) are indicated in addition to the antidepressant treatment.

In cases of depression with suicidality that are extremely difficult to treat by other means, electroconvulsive therapy[8] should also be considered, especially because of the rapid onset of action in comparison with antidepressants. Electroconvulsive therapy is also an important option in patients who are refractory to antidepressant treatment.[9]

Unipolar and bipolar depression is usually recurrent. Thus, in patients who have had two or more recurrent episodes, treatment is required to prevent relapse subsequent to acute and maintenance treatment. Antidepressants or lithium are candidates for preventing relapse in unipolar depression. In bipolar depression, lithium is the first choice; carbamazepine and valproate are alternatives in special indications, such as resistance to lithium treatment or lithium intolerance. Of great interest is the increasingly confirmed result that prophylactic treatment with lithium reduces the well-known excess mortality of patients with unipolar or bipolar depression (e.g. a lifetime risk of suicide is about 15% for unipolar depression and 20% for bipolar disorder) to within the normal range. This effect is apparently not only due to the reduction of depressive relapses and related suicidal behaviour but also seems to be the consequence of a direct effect on suicidal behaviour itself.[10,11]

Attention should be paid to two additional problems when antidepressants are given to suicidal depressives. First, immediate antidepressant therapy is contraindicated in cases of intoxication with psychotropic substances (e.g. in an attempted suicide). In case of need, the fading period of intoxication should be bridged with low-potency neuroleptics. Secondly, an increase in drive or normalization of reduced drive often occurs during antidepressant treatment before brightening of mood (so-called drive–mood dissociation). This may require a temporary prescription or a dose increase of a concomitant sedative medication until mood starts to brighten, in order to counteract the increased risk of acting on suicide impulses.

Schizophrenia

Suicidality associated with a schizophrenic psychosis often requires medication in addition to the standard treatment of the schizophrenic symptoms, especially in cases of severe anxiety or excitation. Low-potency neuroleptics are mostly used in these cases (e.g. levomepromazine or thioridazine), owing to their additional antipsychotic effects, whereas tranquillizers are at most administered as adjuvants or in the case of contraindication to neuroleptics. If high doses (e.g. 100 mg levomepromazine intramuscularly or 200 mg thioridazine) are initially required to achieve adequate sedation, special attention must be paid to the risk of acute hypotension with tendency to collapse, particularly directly after standing up.

A different approach is required for suicidal schizophrenic patients who have depressive or negative symptoms. If depressive–apathetic symptoms with suicidality exist as part of a postpsychotic depression or a deficit syndrome, pharmacotherapy should generally follow the guidelines for the treatment of these conditions. This means that treatment with antidepressants in the case of postpsychotic depression and treatment with atypical neuroleptics or SSRIs (or both) in the deficit syndrome is necessary. If the suicidal symptoms are a side effect of neuroleptic treatment (pharmacogenic depression or akinesia), the neuroleptic dose should be reduced if possible or an antiparkinson drug such as biperiden administered in addition.

References

1. Möller HJ. Steinmeyer EM. Are serotonergic reuptake inhibitors more potent in reducing suicidality? An empirical study on paroxetine. *Eur Neuropsychopharmacol* 1994;**4**:55–59.

2. Möller HJ. Effectiveness and safety of benzodiazepines. *J Clin Psychopharmacol* 1999; **19(Suppl 2):**2–11.

3. Kapfhammer HP, Hippius H. Special feature: pharmacotherapy in personality disorders. *J Pers Disord* 1998;**12**:277–288.

4. Möller HJ. Provocation of aggressive and autoaggressive behavior by psychoactive drugs. *Eur Neuropsychopharmacol* 1994;**4**:232–234.

5. Montgomery SA, Montgomery DB, Green M, et al. Pharmacotherapy in the prevention of suicidal behavior. *J Clin Psychopharmacol* 1992;**12(Suppl 2):** 27S–31S.

6. Möller HJ. Antidepressants: do they decrease or increase suicidality? *Pharmacopsychiatry* 1992; **25**:249–253.

7. Möller HJ, Volz HP. Drug treatment of depression in the 1990s. An overview of achievements and future possibilities. *Drugs* 1996; **52**:625–638.

8. Fink M. Convulsive therapy: theory and practice. Raven: New York; 1979.

9. Möller HJ. Non-response to antidepressants: risk factors and therapeutic possibilities. *Int Clin Psychopharmacol* 1994;9 **(Suppl 2):**17–23.

10. Thies-Flechtner K, Muller-Oerling-hausen B, Seibert W, et al. Effect of prophylactic treatment on suicide risk in patients with major affective disorders. Data from a randomized prospective trial. *Pharmacopsychiatry* 1996;**29:**103–107.

11. Muller-Oerlinghausen B, Berghofer A. Antidepressants and suicidal risk. *J Clin Psychiatry* 1999; **60(Suppl 2):**94–99.

Section VI
Special topics: the young and elderly

21
Adolescent suicide and attempted suicide

Alan Apter

Introduction

Epidemiology

Violence is by far the most common cause of death in young people. This may take the form of suicide, homicide or motor vehicle accidents. Different countries have different rates of each of these phenomena; in most countries suicide rates are higher than homicide rates, and in many industrialized nations the number of young people dying from suicide is higher than the number of fatalities from road accidents. Moreover, in the past two decades motor accident fatalities have been decreasing while suicide, especially among young males, has been increasing. Thus youth suicide poses a major public health problem.

In addition to deaths among young people from suicide, many young people make non-fatal deliberate attempts to kill themselves. This phenomenon (also known as 'attempted suicide', 'parasuicide' or 'deliberate self harm') is at least 10–100 times more common than suicide, although the exact prevalence of such acts is unknown. The relationship between attempted suicide (parasuicide) and suicide is controversial but non-fatal suicidal behaviour remains an acute clinical problem.

A massive increase in the numbers of young people in the West who take intentional overdoses or deliberately injure themselves has been observed. As a result, deliberate self-poisoning has become the most common reason for acute hospital admission among adolescent women. Most statistics on attempted suicide (parasuicide) are derived from hospital samples, which represent only about one-third of actual attempted suicides. Attempted suicide (parasuicide) is more common in females than in males, the sex ratio being highest during adolescence. The highest rates for females are in the age range of 15–19 years. Rates of attempted suicide are inversely related to social class.[1-3]

Reasons for the increases in suicidal behaviour

Theories on the recent outbreak of suicidality have focused on those countries with the most dramatic increases in youth suicide such as Ireland. The rise in suicide among young males in Ireland has paralleled increases in the rates of illegitimacy, crime, alcoholism and unemployment and a decrease in the marriage rate. Other social factors that correlate with youth suicide are a high divorce rate, a low number of nuclear families, high unemployment, high homicide rates, increased number of women in employment or at university and diminishing church membership.[2,4]

Furthermore, there have been striking changes in the nature of adolescence over recent decades. There has been a decrease in the age at which the biological manifestations of puberty occur. For example, menarche in the West used to be at the age of 16–18 years; today it is closer to 12–13 years. Thus, biological changes occur at a much earlier age, an age at which the adolescent is not psychologically and cognitively able to deal with these challenges.

The psychosocial moratorium, as described by Erikson, means that adolescence is greatly prolonged in today's Western society. The age at which young people have to commit themselves to marriage and children as well as a definite career has been greatly increased. There are also more leeways for experimentation with different identities, such as homosexuality, bisexuality[5] and delinquency. This psychosocial moratorium is important for the development of complex industrial societies but takes its toll on the psychic endurance and stable identity of youth.[6]

The role of neurobiological factors is described in Chapter 3.

Risk factors for youth suicide

One of the major risk factors for youth suicide is the presence of a diagnosable psychiatric disorder, especially affective disorder and borderline personality disorder. As in adults, attempted suicide is an important risk factor for suicide.[2,7]

Borderline personality disorder is traditionally associated with non-fatal suicide attempts but there is increasing evidence that suicide is common in these patients as well. Intentional self-damaging acts and suicide attempts are the 'behavioural speciality' of these patients. About 9% of patients with borderline personality disorder eventually kill themselves.[8]

Former adolescent psychiatric patients are at special risk of eventual suicide (10% for males and 1% for females). A family history of psychiatric disorder is also common (25–50 per cent) in adolescent suicide victims, as is the presence of substance or alcohol abuse (33–70 per cent). The comorbidity of affective disorder, personality disorder and substance abuse is especially lethal. The presence of firearms in the home and issues of gender identity such as homosexuality are also well-recognized risk factors for adolescent suicide.[9]

Four co-morbid constellations can be identified as having special significance for suicide in adolescent populations:

- the combination of schizophrenia, depression and substance abuse;
- the combination of substance abuse, conduct disorder and
  depression;
- the combination of affective disorder, eating disorder and anxiety
  disorders; and
- the combination of affective disorder, personality disorder (cluster A,
  paranoid and schizoid personality disorder, in the terminology of the
  Diagnostic and Statistical Manual of Mental Disorders (DSM)) and
  dissociative disorders (disruption in integrated functions of
  conciousness, memory, identity or perception of the environment).

These constellations require vigorous psychiatric intervention.

Affective disorders

Depression

Among teenagers, both attempted and completed suicide are, in the
great majority of cases, preceded by depressive symptoms. There are
considerable differences between depressed children and young people
who have made suicide attempts and those who have not. Depressed
young people who attempt suicide often come from broken families and
have had one or more relatives who have committed or attempted suicide. They have also, relatively often, run away from home and thus been
brought up without favourable role models. Physical and mental abuse,
as well as sexual assault, are also more common in this group. Young
people who have attempted suicide often have lasting problems at
school and also difficulties in achieving workable relationships with their
peers compared with young people who are depressed and have not
attempted suicide. Abuse of alcohol and drugs, impulsive behaviour and
asocial behaviour are additional risk factors for attempted and completed
suicide among depressed young people.[4,10]

Owing to the high incidence of depression among young people who
have attempted suicide, it is important to make a diagnosis and provide
adequate treatment at an early stage. Studies show that depressive disturbances are more common among children and young people than was
previously believed. Unfortunately, many young people with depression are
not identified, partly because their depressive symptoms are often atypical
and partly because adults do not readily recognize depressive symptoms
in the young, owing to their wish to see their children as happy and healthy.
Since the number of young people with depression appears to have
increased since the Second World War, and the age of onset of depressive

disturbances has decreased, it is important to increase the effort to detect depressions in order to be able to prevent suicidal behaviour.[11]

Major depression is most easily diagnosed when it appears acutely in a previously healthy child; in such cases the symptoms closely resemble those seen in adults (see Chapter 4). Often, however, the onset is insidious and the child may show many other difficulties such as attention deficit disorder or separation anxiety disorder before becoming depressed.

Mood disorders tend to be chronic when they start at an early age and the child comes from a family in which there is a high incidence of mood disorders and alcohol abuse.

In some cases the depressed adolescent may also be psychotic and have hallucinations and delusions, which are usually mood congruent. When the psychotic themes are related to suicide, as occurs in command hallucinations or delusions of guilt, the risk of suicide is very high.[11]

Bipolar disorder

Bipolar disorder was once thought to occur only rarely in youth. However, approximately 20 per cent of all bipolar patients have their first episode during adolescence, with a peak age of onset between 15 and 19 years. Developmental variations in presentation, symptomatic overlap with other disorders and lack of clinician awareness have all led to underdiagnosis or misdiagnosis in children and adolescents. Therefore, clinicians need to be aware of some of the unique clinical characteristics associated with the early-onset form. Similarly, it is important to recognize the various phases and patterns of episodes associated with bipolar disorder. The first presentation may be with either manic or depressive episodes. Between 20 and 30 per cent of young people with major depressions go on to have manic episodes.

Adolescents with bipolar disorder are at increased risk of completed suicide. Twenty per cent of adolescents with bipolar disorder made at least one medically significant suicide attempt. In the literature relating to adults, a large review of studies that examined depressive and manic–depressive disorders found that the mean rate of completed suicides was 19 per cent. Patients who are male or who are in the depressed phase of their illness are at the highest risk.[9,11]

Schizophrenia

Schizophrenia is a common psychiatric disorder of adolescence (hence the term 'dementia praecox'). Because schizophrenia is a serious disorder with ominous prognosis and social stigma, some clinicians are hesitant to make this diagnosis even when there is sufficient evidence to do so. This potentially denies the child and family access to appropriate treatment, knowledge about the disorder and specialized support services. However, despite diagnostic criteria being met, the initial diagnosis may be inaccurate given the overlap in symptoms between schizo-phrenia, affective disorders with psychotic features and, possibly, per-sonality and dissociative disorders.

The differentiation between schizophrenia, psychotic depression or mania and schizoaffective disorder is not always easy in adolescence, and many conceptual and nosological issues remain to be decided. The patient must then be followed longitudinally, with periodic diagnostic reassessments, to ensure accuracy. Patients and families should be edu-cated about these diagnostic issues.

The depression in schizophrenia may be related to the fact that the young person feels that he or she is 'falling apart' and becoming mentally ill, and there is indeed evidence that suicidality and depression in these patients is related to good premorbid function, better insight, higher intel-ligence and preservation of cognitive function. Postpsychotic depression and depressive states caused by neuroleptic medications may also have a role to play in this dangerous condition.

Many schizophrenic patients are depressed and suicidal, especially if they are young and have not been ill for a long time. At least two-thirds of the suicides are related to depression and only a small minority to the psychotic symptoms such as command hallucinations. The suicide often occurs shortly after discharge and thus may be related to lack of social support.

Finally many adolescents with schizophrenia also abuse drugs and alcohol, thus increasing their risk of suicide. Sometimes the abuse is an attempt at self-medication. Anticholinergic medications given for the relief of extrapyramidal symptoms give some adolescent patients a 'high' to which they become addicted, and some patients may simulate extrapyra-midal symptoms in order to obtain these drugs. Child-onset and adoles-cent schizophrenia are often preceded by difficulties of attention and learning, for which stimulant medications are given. In the context of a developing schizophrenic condition there is, again, a potential for abuse and drug-induced depression.[9]

Alcohol and drug abuse

Adolescents with psychoactive substance abuse disorder (PSUD), espe-cially males, are more likely to commit suicide with guns than other ado-lescents. Adolescent suicide also seems to be related to more chronic PSUD in subjects who have not sought treatment. In one study PSUD was typically present for at least 9 years before the suicide.

Intoxication for the purpose of self-medication of anxiety and despon-dency, which often follows a crisis, may trigger suicide in an adolescent who feels shame, humiliation or frustration. It has been suggested that adolescents may use psychoactive substances to bolster their courage to carry out the suicide attempt or suicide. Intoxication may also lead to impaired judgement and decreased inhibition and may thus facilitate suicidal behaviour.[1]

Eating disorders

There has been recent recognition of the very definite increased risk of suicide in girls with eating disorders such as anorexia and bulimia.

Psychological characteristics of adolescent suicide attempters

Impulsivity

An important finding is that of Shaffer et al., who found that a combination of depressive symptoms and antisocial behaviour was the most common antecedent of teenage suicide. 'Assaultiveness' and instability of affect as reflected in borderline personality disorder may also be important correlates of adolescent suicidal behaviour, especially in combination with depression. Impulsivity has frequently been described as a risk factor for suicide and a personality characteristic of adolescent suicide attempters. Lack of impulse control has been found to distinguish adolescent suicide attempters from adolescents with an acute illness. However, impulsivity does not seem to characterize all suicide attempters, since group comparisons have found no difference between suicidal patients and controls on measures of cognitive impulsivity. Instead, impulsivity may be important in identifying high-risk subgroups.[7]

Anger

Several authors have indicated that anger is an emotional state that is often associated with adolescent suicide attempts. Suicide attempters in the emergency room report intense anger before the attempt, and adolescent suicide attempters often exhibit a wide range of aggressive behaviours. However, there has been very little empirical investigation of this subject. Pfeffer has described an angry assaultive subtype of childhood suicidal behaviour, and angry feelings are common in children referred for psychiatric evaluation, including those who are non-suicidal.[12]

Anxiety

Anxiety has been identified as an important risk factor for suicidal behaviour in adolescents. Compared with psychiatric out-patients, suicide attempters exhibit higher levels of anxiety. In a large community sample of adolescents,[13] a significant association between anxiety disorders and suicide attempts was found in males but not in females. A study of Dutch adolescents found that suicide attempters (half of them psychiatric patients and half high-school students) exhibited significantly higher levels of state and trait anxiety than non-depressed non-attempters (the high-school students).

Psychodynamic aspects of adolescent suicide

We live in a world in which we are faced everywhere with evidence of conflict. Humans live in a dangerous world surrounded by sickness and accident, beasts and bacteria, the malignant forces of nature and the vengeful hands of their fellows. One would expect that in the face of these overwhelming blows from all sides, people would unite in a universal brotherhood of beleaguered humanity. However, this is not so. Instead we are faced with an enemy behind the lines, for one of the forces that threatens our existence is self-destruction, that extraordinary propensity of human beings to join hands with external forces in the attack upon their own existence. People say that they want life, liberty and happiness, and yet they sacrifice themselves to injure others and expend time, trouble and energy to shorten the lives of others. Moreover, there are some who, as if lacking something else to destroy, turn their weapons upon themselves. Such observations led to Freud's formulation of the death instinct, a strong impulse to self-destruction that exists from birth in all people. This impulse may lead to suicide in exceptional cases only, as it is opposed by a parallel constructive life force within the personality.

Psychoanalytic theory hypothesizes that, in the unconscious, it is possible to regard one's body as not being part of one and it is also possible to treat the body as if it included the body of someone else. This latter phenomenon is called introjection because a person with whom the individual identifies very much appears to be introjected into the self. Therefore, any desired treatment of the other person can now be carried out upon oneself. This turning back of hostile feelings on the self thus serves the psychological usefulness of displacing unacceptable wishes onto the self (i.e. 'kicking the cat' with one's own body).[14,15] Menninger proposed that a dynamic triad underlies all aggressive behaviour, whether directed inwards or outwards: the wish to die, the wish to kill and the wish to be killed. Thus, many suicides in adolescents represent a revenge on parents since the adolescent was too afraid or felt too guilty to kill someone else.[14]

One of the important dynamics in adolescent suicide is narcissistic injury, in which even a 'cry for help' is felt to be unacceptable to the ego ideal. A recent report on a psychological autopsy of 18–21-year-old male soldiers noted that many of the inexplicable suicides occurred among the most highly functional and successful youngsters, who had committed suicide after the most minimal failures. In addition, many of these youngsters were described as being very 'private' people for whom the 'stiff upper lip' code did not allow complaints or requests for help. 'Crying for help' may be more acceptable for girls, and this may partly explain why attempted suicide is more common in girls and completed suicide is more common in boys.[16]

Clinical assessment of suicidal risk

Suicidal adolescents should undergo a comprehensive psychiatric and psychological evaluation. It may be advisable to hospitalize most attempters to reinforce the seriousness of the problem to the child and the family and to ensure evaluation, since lack of compliance with treatment is characteristic of suicidal adolescents who are brought to emergency rooms.

Often what appears at first to be an impulsive over-reaction to a transient interpersonal problem turns out, on more thorough evaluation, to be symptomatic of more chronic difficulties. An attempt of low lethality may be more indicative of miscalculation than of low intent, so it is important to assess what result the child expected. A child with low intent or attention-seeking motives may be at higher risk as a result of impulsivity or a miscalculation in the direction of higher lethality.

In young people, in whom assessment takes time, emergency room personnel tend to take a rapid history of present circumstances and briefly assess for depression, and the mistaken diagnosis of adjustment disorder is often made. A careful history of impulsive behaviour and conduct problems should be taken. This is especially important in adolescents who are identified as being school drop-outs, truants or unemployed. A history of drug and alcohol use as well as questions of identity and sexual orientation[5] must be sought in all patients.

Because suicidal intent is often secretive in nature, it is critically important to establish rapport during the initial interview. Children and adolescents are more likely to respond to an active and responsive clinician. Although confidentiality may be a concern, it is wise to avoid promises of blanket confidentiality. Discussing with the child ahead of time what will be discussed with parents and, if possible, having the child present during the discussion with the parents helps maintain rapport and increases the chance of future compliance. Delineating specifically what further evaluation or treatment modality will address the problem can increase compliance. Because about half of suicide attempters fail to keep their first appointment, having the child and family meet the future therapist and having an appointment made for them may improve the attrition rate.

In addition to asking about suicidal intent, attitude towards death, recent stressors, availability of suicidal means, level of protection at home, the presence or absence of previous attempts and exposure to suicide, psychiatric diagnoses require systematic evaluation. The symptoms associated with major depressive disorder, bipolar disorder, oppositional-defiant disorder (especially with impulsivity and aggression), substance or alcohol abuse and psychosis should be assessed. The presence or absence of these symptoms, as well as the youngster's psychological and psychodynamic personality structure, is important in formulating a treatment plan.[1,12,17–19]

Treatment

Treatment must encompass the acute management of suicidal behaviour as well as treatment of associated mental disorders.[18,19]

Acute management

A major problem in the management of adolescent suicide attempters[1,4,17,20,21] is the failure of adolescent attempters to attend and complete treatment. It has been suggested that about half of the adolescent suicide attempters do not receive adequate psychotherapy after their attempt. Parental denial and psychopathology may interfere with treatment planning. Some clinicians have attempted to deal with this problem by mandating the admission of all adolescent suicide attempters to a general hospital for brief therapy and evaluation. This policy has been widely adopted and has recently been made compulsory by law in Israel.

Since family relationship difficulties are extremely common in adolescent attempters, one might expect that family therapy would be the most productive way of helping suicidal youngsters. This approach appears, however, to be severely limited in effectiveness in many cases because of the high rejection rate by parents, as reflected by high levels of non-attendance at treatment sessions.

Recently, several experts have tried to develop systematic 'manualized' therapies for adolescent suicide attempters based on evidence that shows deficiencies of problem-solving abilities in adolescents shortly after the attempt. Some of these therapies have been shown to be of value in randomized controlled trials.[21–23]

Hospitalization

Clinicians should be prepared to hospitalize suicide attempters who express a persistent wish to die or who are psychiatrically ill until their mental state or level of suicidal behaviour has stabilized.[17] A relationship with the suicidal adolescent and his family should be established in the emergency room and the importance of treatment should be stressed. An appointment and a follow-up plan should be scheduled before discharge. A 'no-suicide contract', in which the child or adolescent agrees not to engage in self-harming behaviour and to tell an adult if he or she is having suicidal urges, may be useful but should not be relied on. The contract should never decrease a clinician's vigilance or curtail monitoring of the child or adolescent. Clinicians should also be aware of suicide contagion in the case of exposure to suicidal behaviour on a ward (see Chapter 31).

Discharge home

Suicidal adolescents should only be discharged home if the clinician is satisfied that adequate supervision and support will be available over the next few days and if a responsible adult has agreed to dispose of potentially lethal medications and firearms. It is valuable for the clinician to warn the child or adolescent and the parents about the dangerous disinhibiting effects of alcohol and other drugs.

The clinician treating the suicidal child or adolescent during the days after an attempt should be available to the patient and family, have experience managing suicidal crises and have support available for him or herself.

Once a therapeutic alliance is established and the child or adolescent has attended the first treatment sessions, the child or adolescent is more likely to continue treatment. Length of the treatment is individual, but 3–6 months should be a rule, with successively fewer contacts up to 1 or 2 years, sometimes longer.[1,23]

Long-term treatment management

Psychotherapy

Psychotherapy, an important component of treatment for the mental disorders associated with suicidal behaviour, should be tailored to the particular needs of the patient. Cognitive– behavioural therapy,[21] interpersonal therapy,[24] dialectical behavioural therapy,[8] psychodynamic therapy[25] and family therapy[23] are all options.

Psychopharmacology

Any medication prescribed to the suicidal child or adolescent must be carefully monitored by a third party and any change of behaviour or side effects should be reported immediately.[26]

Lithium

Lithium greatly reduces the rate of both suicides and suicide attempts in adults with bipolar disorder. Discontinuing lithium treatment in bipolar patients is associated with an increase in suicide morbidity and mortality. Clinical guidelines on the optimum treatment strategies for bipolar adolescents have been established.

Antidepressants

Tricyclic antidepressants should not be prescribed for the suicidal child or adolescent as a first line of treatment. They are potentially lethal, because of the small difference between therapeutic and toxic levels of the drug, and they have not been proved effective in children or adolescents.

Selective serotonin reuptake inhibitors (SSRIs) reduce suicidal ideation and suicide attempts in non-depressed adults with cluster-B (borderline, antisocial, histrionic, narcissistic) personality disorders. They are safe in children and adolescents, have low lethality and are effective in treating depression in non-suicidal adolescents. Further research is needed to determine whether SSRIs influence suicidal behaviour or ideation in children and adolescents. Since SSRIs may have a disinhibiting effect (especially in patients with SSRI-induced akathisia — subjective restlessness accompanied by observed different kinds of movement) and increase suicidal ideation in a small number of adults who were not previously suicidal, children and adolescents prescribed SSRIs must be carefully monitored to ensure that any new suicidal ideation or akathisia is noted.

Anxiolytics
Other medications that may increase disinhibition or impulsivity, such as the benzodiazepines and phenobarbital, should be prescribed with caution in children and adolescents.

Case history

John was a 17-year-old boy who was admitted to an adolescent unit after swallowing 20 pills of fluoxetine, which he had been taking for depression. He reported being depressed for as long as he could remember. As a child he had been obese and was frequently the object of ridicule from his schoolmates. In addition he suffered from a learning disability, which greatly distressed his parents who had hoped that this intelligent child would be a source of pride to them. This was especially a blow to his father, who was a computer technician and was frustrated by his own failure to become an engineer. At an early age John developed symptoms of oppositional disorder. He was disobedient at school and would talk back to his parents at home. He got into frequent fights with his younger brother, who suffered from attention deficit disorder and also had a short temper. As he approached puberty, John's conduct began to get worse. He started to steal and to lie and to write graffiti all over his school and also to vandalize property. He began to smoke heavily and would often play truant from school. He managed to lose weight and became an attractive youngster; however, he still regarded himself as ugly and had a poor self-image. Several attempts at psychological treatment failed, owing to his lack of compliance. At about the age of 13 years he began to drink alcohol and smoke marijuana. In addition he would also get 'high' on solvents. At the age of 14 years he began to write poetry and songs, all of which were pervaded by themes of death and suicide. He would listen for hours to music, especially heavy metal and 'trash'. He identified with Kurt Cobain's suicide and also with the suicide of a friend at school. The final trigger for his suicide attempt was a break-up with his girlfriend.

On examination he was dishevelled, with long hair and many ear-rings, and he was defiant and angry and very obviously depressed. The main theme of his thought was hatred towards his parents, especially his father. He dismissed his mother as 'irrelevant'.

The unit diagnoses were 'double' depression (dysthymia and recurrent major depressive disorder), conduct disorder, substance abuse, attention deficit disorder and developmental reading disorders. In addition, he was thought to have a borderline personality disorder.

Surprisingly, he made good progress on the unit and developed a close relationship with his therapist, a psychiatric resident. However, when the resident had to leave the unit and go to another rotation, John became very angry and upset and decided to discharge himself. Attempts at rehabilitation were at first promising but his drug habit got worse and he started to use hallucinogens in order to self-medicate his depression. He then asked to return to the in-patient unit. Once again there was a period of progress until one day while at home on leave he had an argument with his mother and then another argument with his girl-friend. He took a large dose of lysergic acid diethylamide (LSD) and threw himself out of a fifth storey window of his home.

This case illustrates many of the risk factors that are relevant to adolescent suicide – the presence of mental illness, alcohol and drug abuse, conduct disorder and poor communication within the family. In addition, the presence of a personality disorder and lack of compliance with therapy may be due to disappointment made this case all the more difficult to treat.

References

1. American Academy of Child and Adolescent Psychiatry. Practice parameters for the assessment and treatment of children and adolescents with depressive disorders. *J Am Acad Child Adolesc Psychiatry* 1998;**37(Suppl 10):** 63S–83S.

2. Diekstra RF. The epidemiology of suicide and parasuicide. *Acta Psychiatr Scand* 1993;**371(suppl):** 9–20.

3. Fergusson DM, Lynskey MT. Suicide attempts and suicidal ideation in a birth cohort of 16-year-old New Zealanders. *J Am Acad Child Adolesc* Psychiatry 1995;**34:**1308–1317.

4. Clark D. Suicidal behavior in childhood and adolescence: recent studies and clinical implications. *Psychiatr Ann* 1993;**23:** 271–283.

5. Garofalo R, Wolf RC, Wissow LS, et al. Sexual orientation and risk of suicide attempts among a representative sample of youth. *Arch Pediatr Adolesc Med* 1999; **153:**487–493.

6. Erikson EH. Identity and the life cycle. New York: WW Norton; 1980.

7. Shaffer D, Gould MS, Fisher P, et al. Psychiatric diagnosis in child and adolescent suicide. *Arch Gen Psychiatry* 1996;**53:**339–348.

8. Linehan MM. Cognitive behavior therapy of borderline personality disorder. New York: Guilford Press; 1993.

9. Marttunen M, Aro H, Henriksson M, Lönnqvist J. Mental disorders in adolescent suicide. DSM-III-R

axes I and II diagnoses in suicides among 13- to 19-year-olds in Finland. *Arch Gen Psychiatry* 1999;**48:**834–839.

10. Brent DA, Perper JA, Moritz G, et al. Psychiatric risk factors for adolescent suicide: a case-control study. *J Am Acad Child Adolesc Psychiatry* 1993;**32:**521–529.

11. Gould MS, King R, Greenwald S, et al. Psychopathology associated with suicidal ideation and attempts among children and adolescents. *J Am Acad Child Adolesc Psychiatry* 1998;**37:** 915–923.

12. Pfeffer CR. The suicidal child. New York: Guilford Press; 1986.

13. Ohring R, Apter A, Ratzoni G, et al. State and trait anxiety in adolescent suicide attempters. *J Am Acad Child Adolesc Psychiatry* 1996;**35:**154–157.

14. Menninger KA. Man against himself. New York: Harcourt, Brace and Company; 1938.

15. King RA, Apter A. Psychoanalytic perspectives on adolescent suicide. *Psychoanal Study Child* 1996;**51:** 491–511.

16. Apter A, Bleich A, King RA et al. Death without warning? A clinical postmortem study of suicide in 43 Israeli adolescent males. *Arch Gen Psychiatry* 1993;**2:**138–42.

17. Brent DA. The aftercare of adolescents with deliberate self-harm. *J Child Psychol Psychiatr Allied Disciplines* 1997;**38:** 277–286.

18. Rotheram-Borus MJ, Piacentini J, Van Rossem R, et al. Enhancing treatment adherence with a specialized emergency room program for adolescent suicide attempters. *J Am Acad Child Adolesc Psychiatry* 1996;**35:** 654–663.

19. Spirito A. Individual therapy techniques with adolescent suicide attempters. *Crisis* 1997;**18:**62–64.

20. Berman AL, Jobes DA. Treatment of the suicidal adolescent. Death Studies 1994;**18:**375–389.

21. Brent DA, Holder D, Kolko D, et al. A clinical psychotherapy trial for adolescent depression comparing cognitive, family, and supportive therapy. *Arch Gen Psychiatry* 1997;**54:**877–885.

22. Kruesi MJ, Grossman J, Pennington JM, et al. Suicide and violence prevention: parent education in the emergency department. *J Am Acad Child Adolesc Psychiatry* 1999;**38:**250–255.

23. Harrington R, Kerfoot M, Dyer E, et al. Randomized trial of a home-based family intervention for children who have deliberately poisoned themselves. *J Am Acad Child Adolesc Psychiatry* 1998; **37:**512–518.

24. Mufson L, Weissman MM, Moreau D, Garfinkel R. Efficacy of interpersonal psychotherapy for depressed adolescents. *Arch Gen Psychiatry* 1999;**56:**573–579.

25. Kernberg P. Psychological interventions for the suicidal adolescent. *Am J Psychother* 1994;**48:** 52–63.

26. Montgomery SA, Montgomery D. Pharmacological prevention of suicidal behaviour. *J Affect Disord* 1982;**4:**291–298.

22
The elderly and suicide

Diego De Leo and Gaia Meneghel

Introduction

In almost all countries that transmit their demographic statistics to the World Health Organization, older adults present higher suicide rates than young people and, generally, lifetime suicide risk and the wish to die are positively correlated with increase in age.[1,2] People's thoughts about suicide in later life differ from their thoughts about suicide in youth. There is still a tendency to rationalize suicidal ideation and behaviour in the elderly and to consider self-injury as the result of a well-pondered assessment of the pros and cons of old age. Suicide is, instead, just as irrational a choice for the elderly as for any other age group and is a response to marked psychological distress, conditioned by the presence of psychiatric disorders and poor living conditions, which may render elderly people more vulnerable as a result of physical illness, solitude and feelings of worthlessness.

Epidemiology and special characteristics of suicidal behaviour in the elderly

Fatal suicidal behaviour

Despite tremendous cultural variability across nations, suicide rates are ubiquitously higher among the elderly, although they differ from nation to nation. In Europe, the mean elderly suicide rate for the 5-year period from 1989 to 1993 stood at 29.3 per 100,000.[3] Over the same period in the USA, the rate was 19.7 per 100,000 (versus 14.9 per 100,000 in adults aged 25–44 years).[4] In 1991 in Japan, 45 per cent of female suicides across all ages were by women aged 65 years and over.[5] Suicide is most prevalent among the 'old old' and tends to be more prevalent among men, particularly in the Western world.[6] This contrasts with the objectively poor health and social status experienced by elderly women everywhere that results from poor psychophysical health secondary to greater longevity, poverty, widowhood and abandonment.[7] Protective factors appear to be:

- a greater capacity to adjust than men;
- preservation of a better-established social network;
- greater self-sufficiency in activities of daily living; and
- strengthened feelings of usefulness through commitment to children and grandchildren.

Suicide methods in the elderly are generally violent (even among women), expressing high suicidal intention. The most common self-destructive methods are by firearms (particularly in the USA), hanging, jumping from high places, self-poisoning (especially with medicines such as benzodiazepines and analgesics among women) and drowning.[5,8]

Summer appears to be the highest-risk season for elderly suicide, with its high humidity and – in continental climates – its torrid daylight hours (an association possibly governed by the interaction of biological and social factors).[8]

In most cases, old-age suicide takes place in the elderly person's home, in solitude. Suicide notes are less frequently left by older adults and, when present, disclose determination, clear intent, reflection and emotional detachment.[4]

Although contacts with a medical practitioner before suicide are frequent among the elderly, they tend to be non specific and, perhaps, not sufficiently regular. Findings indicate that 90 per cent of suicide victims aged over 65 years had seen their general practitioner in the 3 months before death and that 50 per cent had seen their general practitioner during the final week of life. Psychiatric consultation had been requested in only about 20–25 per cent of suicides. In these cases, only one-fifth of elderly patients verbalized death thoughts and suicide intent. In particular, men and attempted suicide repeaters were poor communicators.[4]

Non-fatal suicidal behaviour

Attempted suicides (parasuicide) are rare among the elderly but, when present, they are a very important indicators of suicide risk. They are four times less frequent among elderly women than young women, and three times less frequent among elderly men than young men.[9] The ratio of parasuicide to suicide among the elderly is 2.09:1,[3] which differs greatly from the ratio in the general population (between 8:1 and 20:1).[10] Older persons are less likely to have made a previous attempt (in 33 per cent of cases) than younger persons (50 per cent). Parasuicide is more prevalent among the 'young old' and especially among women.[10]

The low parasuicide rate among the elderly may be explained by a greater desire to die and determination that the act should end fatally.

Parasuicides may be considered 'failed' suicides rather than a 'cry for help', unlike the situation for many young people. This confers a more negative prognostic value on the presence of a previous parasuicide in a patient's history compared with other age groups. On the basis of this finding, it has also been argued that studying parasuicide in the elderly might allow us to develop a clearer understanding of suicide and its prevention than in other ages.

Death thoughts and suicide intentionality have been reported to be present in the elderly population at frequencies of 15.9% and 2.3%, respectively, according to the various samples and time periods surveyed.[11] The age bands most highly affected are the 'oldest old' (85 years and over) and women.[11]

Since the vast majority of elderly suicides do not present a history of previous suicidal behaviour, detection and management of those with suicide ideation may assume special importance. Nonetheless, while ideation has emerged as an important predictor of self-destruction, identification of these subjects is hindered by the presence of several confounders, such as anhedonia, tiredness of life, and the wish to be dead. At the present time, it remains unclear whether these mentioned factors are distinct phenomena or different levels of severity of a single phenomenon.

Estimates and underestimates of suicidal behaviour in the elderly

Underestimation of the suicide phenomenon among the elderly is particularly frequent. Deaths by suicide may not be reported as such to the authorities by relatives for cultural reasons (e.g. fear of reproach) or insurance purposes. In other situations, suicide is not recorded since it is not recognized as such and death is attributed to accidental or natural causes. This applies in particular to ambiguous road accidents or domestic deaths for which there is a greater tendency to believe that an elderly person was seized by a sudden, unforseeable illness rather than dying by self-inflicted injury. Other forms of misled suicide are self-inflicted death by indirect methods, such as 'suicidal erosion', which are relatively common among the elderly.[12] Such behaviours take the form of refusal to eat (leading to slow but definite starvation), refusal to use life-sustaining medications (insulin therapy, for example), or sustained use of alcohol and psychotropic drugs. Lastly, those aged over 65 years are the people at highest risk of a prognosis for the somatic consequences of attempted suicide. Hence some deaths are not attributed to previous self-injury, but are imputed to other pathophysiological causes, particularly when a long time elapses between parasuicide and death.

Although the suicide rate in those aged over 75 years is up to seven times higher than the adolescent suicide rate in all continents and the order of magnitude of these indices is stable over a time period of approximately 30 years,[13] some differences in past (and probably future) trends have been observed in countries of different culture.

In Anglo-Saxon countries (particularly the USA, Australia and New Zealand) a decline of over 50 per cent has taken place in elderly suicides, particularly among white males.[6] Explanations may be found in the development of elderly political and social activism, improved social services, changing attitudes toward retirement, increased economic security and better psychiatric care. By contrast, the lack of a culture projected towards old age and specific services for older adults in Latin countries may account for the increase in suicide rates in recent years. Moreover, the recent breakdown in family structure may have provoked a significant decline in 'spontaneous' sources of social support (extended, trigenerational families) in the absence of replacement by 'formal' support or education on coping with age.

There is much uncertainty about projected levels of suicide in the elderly. The above-mentioned cultural differences and attitudes toward ageing may play an important role in the future. The same applies to factors that cannot be predicted, such as future health and disease control, pain management and economic conditions and more effective treatment of mental health problems (particularly depression).

It is nonetheless conceivable that, in view of the 'greying' of the population and the considerable lengthening of life expectancy, the absolute (if not relative) number of elderly suicides is destined to increase. Moreover, it has been predicted that suicide – considered globally – will continue to hold its position among the top 10 causes of burden of disease, with a percentage of total burden slightly higher than in 1990 (2.3 per cent) in the year 2020 (2.4 per cent).[14]

High-risk factors in suicide among the elderly

Psychopathology

Psychiatric illness represents the most important risk factor for suicide among the elderly. Over 75 per cent of elderly victims are reported to present a diagnosis of a psychiatric pathology at the time of death. The majority (50–87 per cent) of elderly suicide victims have depressive illness at the time of death, and this is particularly true among the 'old old'. Bipolar disorder is, however, rare and affective disorders with psychotic symptoms is almost absent.[4,8]

The impact of alcohol abuse on suicide prevalence in older persons is not clear. Alcohol abuse and dependence are present according to different studies in 3–44% of elderly suicide victims, which is higher than in the general population of the same age, and are more common among the 'young old'.[4] The combination of drinking and depression, where drinking is a maladjusted coping mechanism, produces a high suicide risk among elderly alcoholics. Sometimes alcohol is used as a complementary suicide method, to potentiate the action of drugs, or for disinhibition purposes.[10]

A small number of elderly suicide victims are affected by schizophrenia or paraphrenia. The prevalence of these disorders (6–17%) is notably higher than in the general elderly population (0.1%).[4]

The prevalence of anxiety and personality disorders among elderly suicides is not clear. Older subjects with anxiety disorders have been shown to be at high suicide risk, especially in the case of anxiety–depressive syndrome.[4] A psychological autopsy study performed by De Leo in 1997 on 15 in-patient suicides (in general hospital geriatric wards) highlighted that, in most cases, very intense anxiety was present. Furthermore, 12 out of the 15 suicides occurred in the morning, especially early in the morning, when anxiety is generally at peak level.[15]

The frequency of personality disorder is much lower than in young people. Suicides are generally associated with the personality trait 'lower openness to experience' and with an inability to form close relationships, tendency to be helpless and hopeless, inability to tolerate change, inability to express psychological pain verbally, loss of control, feelings of loneliness, despair and dependence on others.[4,8]

Dementia hardly features on the diagnostic list of suicides. Some authors have hypothesized that the presence of confusion may explain some unsuccessful attempted suicides in the elderly and also the fact that, in the early stages of dementia, patients may manifest suicidal ideation, but the presence of cognitive impairment may prevent action being carried out. Indeed, the incidence of suicide among patients with dementia does not exceed that of the general elderly population, even in the early stages of dementia.[16,17] Moreover, in one in-patient study, the association between dementia and not committing suicide approached statistical significance.[4] This may be due to poor patient insight, since awareness is impaired from the very early stages of the disease, especially in patients with marked 'frontal' characteristics.[16]

Physical illness

There is controversy as to the influence exerted by physical illness on suicidal behaviour. Sixty-five per cent of older adults are afflicted by a severe, chronic physical pathology at the time of suicide and 27 per cent suffer from persistent, severe illness.[4] Since these conditions reduce autonomy and impose a new lifestyle, they may induce symptoms of depression, helplessness and hopelessness, and lead to mistrust of certain therapies, particularly among men and the 'old old'. Lack of trust in medical intervention and endless suffering are commonly found in depressed elderly suicides.[4] However, the constant copresence of a structural depressive disorder or other psychiatric pathology (e.g. substance abuse) suggests that physical illness alone cannot bring about suicide outside of a psychopathological context. In particular, the pre-existence of certain personality traits, such as a strong, frustrated need to be active and independent, a history of depression and hostility, or a closed, contemplative character seem to be particularly important in this respect.[10]

The importance of comorbidity of psychic and physical disorders in determining suicidal behaviour has been clearly highlighted in cases of suicide among cancer patients and those who fear illness, thereby partially scaling down the concept that suicide is a 'rational' choice in a physically ill older adult.

Terminal illness and cancer

Recent studies indicate increased suicide rates in cancer patients as a whole, especially in men and in the 2 years immediately after diagnosis. The literature reports that 62.5–85 per cent of cancer suicides meet the Diagnostic and Statistical Manual of Mental Disorders, 4th revision (DSM-IV) criteria for a psychiatric diagnosis such as severe depression, anxiety and thought disorders.[18] It is still unclear whether psychopathology was a primary event triggered by physical illness, a secondary consequence of physical illness, such as organic mood disorders (metastatic or non-metastatic effect) or an adverse effect of pharmacotherapy.

Fear of illness

An important aspect of suicide risk related to physical illness concerns patients' feelings and their fears about their illness, even if they do not have an illness. Irrational fear of illness and disability has characterized some suicides, especially in elderly males, in the absence of pathology. In the psychological autopsy conducted by De Leo et al.[19] on 12 suicide victims who were affected by slightly to moderately impaired vision, fear of losing sight alone induced severe psychological distress, leading to suicide. Fear of cancer as a suicide precipitator is a frequent occurrence. In a psychological autopsy study conducted by Hickey et al.,[18] 12 subjects, whose only apparent worry was the fear of having cancer, had taken their own lives. They were elderly males with no known physical illness or psychiatric history; fear of physical illness clearly suggested a more profound psychological problem. Hence, it is essential to assess patients' medical problems, their subjective experience of illness and, primarily, the meaning that may underlie feelings of fear. Thus, fear of having cancer may have been the outcome of a depressive or an anxiety disorder that has gone unrecognized.

Life conditions and events

Widowed, single or divorced people are over-represented among elderly victims, particularly men.[3] Relatively low suicide rates for married people may reflect not only the companionship of marrlage, but also its outlet for aggressiveness.

Up to 50 per cent of elderly victims, especially women, are reported to live alone and to be lonely.[4] Generally speaking, suicidal elderly people seem to have fewer resources and support and fewer contacts with relatives and friends than their younger counterparts, and to live a more solitary existence.[10] Some authors disagree with this view, maintaining that social isolation and stressful life events are no greater in elderly suicide victims than in young suicide victims, except for the higher presence of bereavements and physical pathology.[8,10] According to these authors, elderly suicide is the expression of a 'narcissistic crisis' caused by an inability to tolerate the accumulation of minor day-to-day failures (the 'wedding cake' model). Consequently, suicidal behaviour is precipitated by minor but coincidental events combined with depressive pathology and substance abuse.[20]

Retirement does not in itself constitute an important suicide risk factor, unless it is abrupt, complete and involuntary, particularly in the case of white 'young old' men and in subjects who lack flexibility in dealing with role change or health and social support and who are unable to adjust to the new lifestyle consequent upon retirement.[10] Conversely, socioeconomic decline does not appear to be as important a risk factor for elderly suicide as it is for younger suicide.[8]

Bereavements very frequently constitute stressful life events in late life, and the death of close relatives and friends is the most important factor in precipitating suicide. Risk has been found to be higher for the death of a spouse, especially when sudden; men were more exposed in this respect. Further risk factors include an ambivalent marital relationship, dependence and the presence of a poor social support network for the survivor, belief in the afterlife and, above all, alcohol abuse or dependence disorder. The risk is particularly high in the first 6 months of bereavement.[5,10]

Analysis of suicidal behaviour among institutionalized elderly has not shown higher suicide rates than in the general population. The institutionalized elderly who most frequently manifested suicidal behaviour were residents of crowded institutes with a high staff turnover.[4] Anticipation of or recent nursing home placement were often the significant factor that led to a suicidal act, particularly among those who were married at the time of their suicide.[10] Many protective factors do, however, seem to curb suicide among institutionalized elderly. Psychogeriatric wards and hospital staff probably offer greater protection, more observation for the elderly and a safe asylum in which to prevent the onset of feelings of solitude. In-patient psychogeriatric treatments are probably also effective in reducing psychopathology and in-patient suicide rates. Risk is further reduced by the high rate of institutionalized patients affected by senile dementia compared with the general population. Lastly, the under-reporting of suicide (especially by indirect and ambiguous methods) and the selection bias for admission (by which patients with previous suicidal attempts may not be welcome as residents) may have made a further contribution.

Biological factors

To date, no research in the literature has specifically studied the biology of late-life suicide. Some considerations may nonetheless be drawn from notions on general biological suicidology and findings on the ageing process.[21,22]

The biological bases of suicidal behaviour are reported to lie in impaired regulation of neurotransmitters and neuroreceptors. Studies on the brain ageing process have indicated that there are alterations in synaptic conduction and neurotransmitter systems, such as a reduction in dopamine and norepinephrine content in various areas of the aged brain and a rise in monoamine oxidase levels. Greater controversy surrounds variations in the elderly serotonergic system, since several studies have shown a significant inverse correlation between age and serotonin levels in some cerebral areas (pons, hypothalamus, substantia nigra and amygdala), while others even point to increased serotonin levels in the medulla oblongata. It could be hypothesized that since there is a natural, age-related decline in the activity of some neurones and neurotransmitter systems, the remaining functional neurones simultaneously activate a process of compensation through feedback stimulation. This compensation progress is probably not sufficient. Older adults' greater vulnerability to depression and, more specifically, to suicidal behaviour may thus depend on a defective compensatory mechanism, which promotes the onset and chronicization of the psychopathological process.

It has also been suggested that impaired regulation of the hypothalamus–pituitary– adrenal axis and alterations in the circadian rhythm, both common in the elderly, may in turn play a part in inducing suicidal behaviour in the elderly.[8]

Intervention and prevention of suicidal behaviour in the elderly

Paradoxically, despite ubiquitous, virtually absent planning of preventive strategies specifically tailored for elderly suicide, there has been a fall in suicide rates in many countries. Theoretically, preventive strategies to reduce suicide in the elderly should acknowledge that suicidal 'careers' in this age group (suicidal ideation leading to suicide attempt leading to suicide) are often atypical and frequently lack a history of attempted suicide.

Primary prevention

Primary prevention should focus on subjects who are currently not feeling suicidal and aim at improving societal quality of life in the elderly, with a view to decreasing the risk that such inclination will afflict them in the future.

Important structural intervention includes improvement in older adults' economic status, establishment of an extensive, outreaching social support network and constant control and improvement of psychophysical health status. Reduction of elderly suicide in some countries by relieving economic distress has been achieved through the introduction of social security programmes, a fall in the percentage of elderly persons living below the poverty line, the development of more flexible retirement schemes for the 'young old' and improved health-care availability.[23] Greater opportunities for peer relations and better access to recreational facilities provide support for urban elderly and facilitate role transitions that are typical of old age, including retirement and children leaving home. Systematic monitoring of physical health for preventive purposes, which requires general practitioners to provide an annual physical and mental examination to all their elderly patients, has been in force in the UK for some years now.[4]

Secondary prevention

The objective of secondary prevention is to identify and treat factors that influence suicidal behaviour. Identifying suicidal ideation among the elderly is a goal of primary importance. General practitioners with superior interview skills, good previous knowledge of both the individual patient and their type of condition, and a favourable attitude towards mental illness are generally better able to detect mental distress.[23] These abilities should be improved by appropriate training and educational programmes, which can be addressed to other health professionals (e.g. nurses and social workers) as well as to general practitioners. Training courses should be cyclical (i.e. repeated yearly) to optimize their effect.[4] They should teach recognition of early and atypical symptoms of elderly psychopathology (particularly male depression) and promote eradication of therapeutic nihilism and old-fashioned fears of psychotropic drugs, thereby permitting adequate treatment of potentially reversible mental illness. Some non-pharmacological approaches to the treatment of senile depression may also be considered, particularly cognitive therapy and interpersonal psychotherapy.[23] Given the frequent presence of physical illness among the suicidal elderly, greater attention should be paid to assessing how the disease is being experienced, to discussing fears and analysing personal resources and the ability to react, and to treating chronic and invalidating pain.

Suicide prevention programmes and general mental health facilities are underutilized by elderly suicide victims. The reasons for this range from poor information on their existence and conviction that these services are costly, to the low credit given by older adults to all types of agency or institution.[10] An attempt to overcome elderly reticence to contact alarm-collecting centres has been through the use of 'centripetous' recruitment programmes. One such experience is the 'Tele-Help/Tele-Check' service, established in the Veneto region of Italy.[24] 'Tele-Help' consists of a portable device that, in the event of an emergency, lets users send alarm signals that activate a pre-established network of assistance and help. In 'Tele-Check', trained staff members contact each client on a twice-weekly basis to monitor their condition through a short, informal interview and to offer emotional support. The client may also contact the centre at any time for any reason. Clients are enrolled in the service at the request of local social workers or general practitioners who identify older adults who need additional home help. Since many of the traditional risk factors for suicide were found in the elderly people who were studied, this service appears to provide support of great importance for elderly suicide prevention. This finding, 10 years after the introduction of the service to a population of 20,000 elderly people living at home, has continued to be associated with a statistically significant fall in the number of expected deaths by suicide.

In addition to attendance at more traditional mental health services, the propagation of crisis intervention centres specifically for the aged have proved very effective since they are organized according to the real needs of this population and improve quality of assistance.[12] Good results have been achieved in the USA, with the establishment of help lines operating round the clock.[10] In addition to providing psychological support and telematic services, home visits are provided to frail, isolated and homebound elderly, with a view to reducing isolation and recognizing cries for help. It has been suggested that the elderly, particularly those who live alone and those who suffer from invaliding pathologies, would benefit above all from face-to-face contact, in both home and institutional settings.[10]

Moreover, publicity campaigns may teach the audience to listen more carefully to signs communicated by older people (depressive symptoms or the wish to die), to be attentive to their behaviour and to be active in response when necessary.[23] More information should be provided on health and social centres and on 'hotlines' that deal specifically with the elderly and can be contacted when help is required.

Available clinical experience and scientific evidence indicate that currently employed strategies produce a more visible effect with women.[24] This may be accounted for by various factors, including women's great propensity to communicate their inner feelings and to receive emotional support. In Western cultures in particular, men are less willing to express their emotions and are probably not truly engagable In therapeutic projects that are based mainly on verbalization of suffering. It is therefore more likely that men at risk are more often underdiagnosed and undertreated, especially by general practitioners, than their female counterparts.[25] The development of crisis intervention techniques that are able to modify the male client environment by obtaining the desired changes or by teaching more adaptive strategies seems, at the moment, to be more promising.

Tertiary prevention

Tertiary prevention consists of management of those who have suffered a loss by suicide. Every suicide by an older adult is cause for distress in an average of six people: spouse, siblings and peers, in addition to children, grandchildren and associated kin.[10] The distress level that bereavement by suicide may cause is not generally the same for everyone.

Intervention targeted at working through the grief process should be addressed to all survivors of elderly suicide, although the most needy have proven to be spouses of the same age, since they, too, may be at high suicide risk.[10] Intervention may be both social and health-oriented. It would be appropriate to provide a social support network to prevent isolation and teach a new lifestyle to overcome the ensuing emptiness.[23] To this end it may be helpful to create self-help and resocialization groups in which the bereaved can discuss and share experiences and feelings in a reassuring, family atmosphere, without shame. On emergence of any frank psychopathological profiles, survivors must be referred to mental health facilities to begin pharmacological therapy or structured, continuative psychotherapy. In referring survivors to the various health and social security facilities, an important role may be played by the general practitioner, who is generally the only professional with whom the elderly are in contact and from whom they actively request help and information.

Case history:
An elderly man's lifeline

At the time of his suicide attempt Mr B, aged 77 years, had been a widower for 3 months. He suffered from a functional disability as a result of the amputation of one leg for an incurable vascular problem. His two daughters both lived in distant cities.

After their mother's death, they had begun devoting a half-day each week to looking after their father. They also arranged for some cleaning and cooking to be carried out by home helps hired through private agencies. In co-operation with the family doctor, after Mr B's serious suicide attempt, they requested urgent installation of the 'Tele-Help/Tele-Check' service in his home.

Mr B attempted suicide by dropping a radio in the bath in an effort to electrocute himself. After 3 weeks in hospital, he was discharged with a prescription for 100 mg sertraline daily and the recommendation that a social worker visit him at home at least once a week.

Mr B has no previous history of psychiatric disorders. A retired blue-collar worker, he has no friends or particular hobbies and spends most of his time watching television. He used to play cards with his wife. He was opposed to the idea of connection to the 'Tele-Help/Tele-Check' service, fearing complete abandonment by his daughters.

In the first month of being connected, he made two emergency calls to the service. In both cases, he expressed strong suicidal ideation. Now that he has been connected to the service for nearly 2 years, Mr B receives an average of three check calls a week from the Tele-Help operator, with whom he has established highly effective and supportive communication.

References

1. Barnow S, Linden M. Suicidality and tiredness of life among very old persons: results from the Berlin Aging Study (BASE). *Arch Suicide Res 1997;**3:**171–182.

2. World Health Organization. World Health Statistics Annual. Geneva: World Health Organization; 1995.

3. De Leo D, Padoani W, Scocco P, et al. Elderly suicidal behaviour: results from the WHO\EURO Multicentre Study on Parasuicide. *Int J Geriat Psychiatry*; in press.

4. Shah AK, De T. Suicide and the elderly. *Int J Psychiatry Clin Pract* 1998;**2:**3–17.

5. McIntosh JL. Suicide prevention in the elderly (age 65–99). *Suicide Life Threat Behav* 1995;**25:** 180–192.

6. De Leo D. Cultural issues in suicide and old age. Crisis 1999; **20:**53–55.

7. Canetto SS. Gender and suicide in the elderly. *Suicide Life Threat Behav* 1992;**22:**80–97.

8. Steffens DC, Blazer DG. Suicide in the elderly. In: Jacobs DG (ed). The Harvard Medical School guide to suicide assessment and intervention. San Francisco: Jossey-Bass Publishers; 1999.

9. Schmidtke A, Bille-Brahe U, De Leo D, et al. Attempted suicide in Europe: rates, trends and sociodemographic characteristics of suicide attempters during the period 1989–1992. Results of the WHO/EURO Multicentre Study on Parasuicide. *Acta Psychiatr Scand* 1992;**93:**327–338.

10. McIntosh JL, Santos JF, Hubbard RW, et al. Elderly suicide research, theory and treatment. Washington, DC: American Psychological Association; 1994.

11. Scocco P, Meneghel G, Dello Buono M, et al. Suicidal ideation and its correlates: survey of an over-65-year-old population. J Nervous Mental D. In press.

12. De Leo D, Diekstra RFW. Depression and suicide in late life. Toronto: Hogrefe and Huber; 1990.

13. Gulbinat W. The epidemiology of suicide in old age. In: Diekstra RFW, Gulbinat W, Kienhorst I et al. (eds). Preventive Strategies on suicide. Leiden, The Netherlands: EJ Brill; 1995:35–49.

14. Murray CJL, Lopez AD. Global

burden of disease and injury series, vol 1. Boston: Harvard University Press; 1996.

15. De Leo D. Note sui comportamenti suicidari di anziani in ospedale generale [Considerations on suicidal behaviour of general hospital elderly inpatients]. *Ital J Suicidol* 1997;**7:** 49–51.

16. De Leo D. Dementia, insight, and suicidal behavior. *Crisis* 1996;**17:** 147–148.

17. Harris EC, Barraclough B. Suicide as an outcome for mental disorders. A meta-analysis. *Br J Psychiatry* 1997;**170:**205–228.

18. Hickey P, Meneghel G, De Leo D, et al. Comparing fear of illness and disability: a psychological autopsy study. Submitted for publication.

19. De Leo D, Hickey P, Meneghel G, et al. Blindness, fear of blindness and suicide. *Psychosomatics* 1999;**40:**339–344.

20. Clark DC. Narcissistic crises of aging and suicidal despair. *Suicide Life Threat Behav* 1993; **23:**21–26.

21. Mann JJ. The neurobiology of suicide. *Nature Med* 1998;**4:**25–30.

22. Rifai AH, Reynolds CF, Mann JJ. Biology of elderly suicide. *Suicide Life Threat Behav* 1992;**22:**49–61.

23. De Leo D, Scocco P. Treatment and prevention of suicidal behaviour in the elderly. In: Hawton K, van Heringen K (eds). Suicide and attempted suicide. Chichester: John Wiley and Sons; 2000.

24. De Leo D, Carollo G, Dello Buono M. Lower suicides rates associated with Tele-Help/Tele-Check service for the elderly at home. *Am J Psychiatry* 1995;**152:** 632–634.

25. Haste F, Charlton J, Jenkins R. Potential for suicide prevention in primary care? *Br J Gen Pract* 1998;**48:**1759–1763.

Section VII
Prevention

VIIA *Health-care perspectives*
VIIB *Public health perspective*

23
Strategy in suicide prevention

Danuta Wasserman

Attitudes towards the suicide-prone person

Suicide is preventable, but different groups of suicidal people require different strategies.[1] Risk factors, risk situations and treatment options have been described in previous chapters. However, it is not enough to convey this knowledge without, at the same time, shedding light on the strong feelings aroused by suicide. These may range from compassion and guilt to fear of, and turning one's back on, people who attempt or commit suicide because the act openly challenges the instinct of self-preservation, which (in most people) is strong.

Many young people and people who have not experienced suicidal thoughts or mental ill-health tend to interpret suicide as an act that expresses both control over one's life situation and freedom. The truth is, however, that most suicidal acts arise in situations in which life is unbearable and everything is perceived as being out of reach of the individual's control. In this kind of situation, philosophical statements about suicide being a human right can seem derisive and uncaring to a person on the brink of suicide, and distressing to the devoted health professional. For a person who lacks knowledge of suicidology, this kind of 'philosophical' attitude may serve as a pretext for not intervening when someone is suicidal, on the grounds that the individual's integrity and right of self-determination should be respected. This kind of view may also make health-care staff passive, with devastating consequences for suicidal patients and their relatives.

Taboos as psychological defence mechanisms

The strong taboo on suicide that still exists and the distress it arouses and has aroused throughout history make it difficult to approach the problem of suicide in an open and scientific way. To this day, suicide is associated with shame, uneasiness and guilt. As a result, suicides are concealed and the view is reinforced of suicide as being predestined and impossible to prevent or treat.

The guilt that we may feel, both individually and collectively, because there are people among us who have no wish to live, contributes to our deafness to suicidal communication and our desire to ward off the knowledge that this communication is in the majority of cases a conscious or unconscious cry for help. Suicidal communication usually brings to the fore in the recipient uncomfortable thoughts about death and the meaning of the life. Keeping at bay problems that evoke strong negative feelings and reflections is a normal psychological defence mechanism. In the bustle of everyday life, the main wish of most people is probably to avoid dealing with it. As professionals, however, we must strive for awareness of the issues raised by suicide and how they affect our work.

Suicide-prevention programmes

The World Health Organization (WHO) and the United Nations have drafted strategy proposals for the work on suicide prevention and there are currently several national programmes for suicide prevention in existence.[2-4] The WHO has published a series of documents on how to prevent suicide in psychiatric and general practice settings, in schools, prisons and in survivors of suicide, as well as documents on how to report suicide in the media.[5]

Strategies in suicide prevention

In suicide prevention work, strategies can be pursued through the health-care services or directed at the general population (Figure 23.1). Although various psychiatric treatments have had the best-documented effects on suicide prevention, the emphasis of work needs shift to an earlier stage of the suicidal process, and it is advisable that both sets of strategies go hand in hand, for maximum overall impact.

Health-care approach

When suicide-prevention efforts are initiated in the population by means of information campaigns, many new individuals or groups in need of help are found. Psychiatric staff may become discontented if they lack the knowledge and resources to provide satisfactory care for those who seek help. Such dissatisfaction may have an adverse impact on suicidal people who, being very fragile, sensitive and thin-skinned, may feel rejected if they meet frustrated staff. Poor care increases the risk of suicidal acts, since it is not only people's propensity to seek and accept help that determines whether their suicidal process can be arrested or whether it culminates in attempted or completed suicide. The course of the suicidal

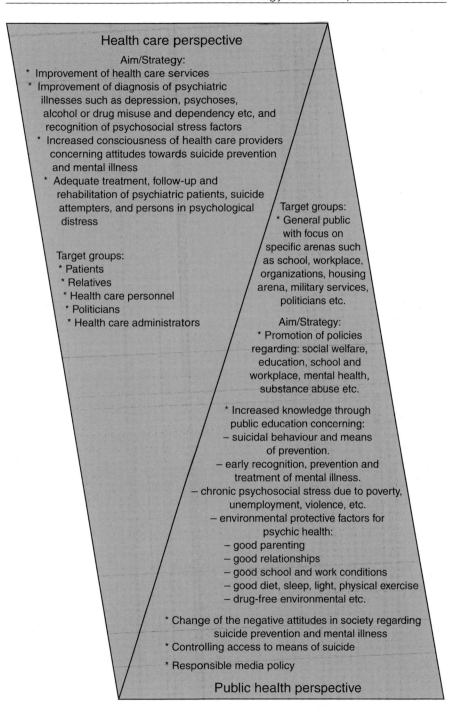

Figure 23.1

Strategies for suicide prevention. Wasserman, 1999.

process also depends on the capacity of others, including care staff, to recognize suicidal people's needs and give them adequate treatment.

Therefore, the work of my group at the Swedish National Centre for Suicide Research and Prevention of Mental Ill-Health, like suicide preventive activities in many other countries, focuses on a risk group-oriented, three-pronged strategy to facilitate the successive development of population-oriented suicide prevention. The strategy consists of:

- identifying risk groups;
- improving the diagnosis and treatment of suicidal patients, including those who have attempted suicide; and
- offering better rehabilitation for suicide attempters.

Adequate treatment of mental illnesses in psychiatric settings and in the general population through the work of general practitioners has hitherto been one of the most thoroughly tried and tested strategies for reducing suicide risk.

Public-health approach

Psychosocial support
Modern society is evolving along paths that give individuals greater responsibility for their own lives and personal development through expanded access to knowledge, mediated in part by the explosive growth of information technology. At the same time, many people are increasingly isolated and lack support in their immediate surroundings. Numerous people are in the throes of existential crisis and, in their loneliness, may find life pointless and see suicide as the only possible way out.

Population-oriented suicide prevention focuses on building up supportive networks and strengthening the life skills that protect people in difficult situations and also on providing close-range support to counteract the isolation felt by susceptible people. The back-up for vulnerable people who need support from others to cope with stress because they lack a network of family and friends is needed in some cases throughout the whole life. This support works best if it is socially and culturally adapted to the recipients' needs.

Public attitudes and knowledge
Changes in attitudes towards people close to suicide and more knowledge about prevention of suicide and mental ill-health are further objectives. In many countries, population-oriented efforts concentrate on children and adolescents because it can be difficult to influence adults and the elderly to change their attitudes, whereas the young are relatively flexible.

Programmes aimed at increasing knowledge of mental health and ill-health and of health-promoting measures attempt to eliminate the fears and misunderstandings that surround suicide. However, there is a degree of risk that poorly devised information inputs may provoke suicidal acts, especially among adolescents and certain sensitive people. Being suggestible, these people may imitate a suicidal behaviour that has taken place in their immediate surroundings or one that has received coverage in the mass media.

It is not wrong to speak and write of suicide, but it must be done in the right way, without glorifying or romanticizing the act or dismissing it as incomprehensible (see also Chapter 31). The difficulties in life that have contributed to suicidal peoples' decisions to take their own lives should be described honestly, without circumvention. Simultaneously, specific and practical examples and options for extricating oneself from a suicidal dilemma should be given. Hushing up the problem, showing ambivalence and turning a blind eye to the subject only strengthen prejudices and reinforce ignorance, thereby leaving suicidal people to cope unaided.

Environmental measures
Population-oriented suicide prevention also includes environmental measures, such as restriction of access to dangerous means of committing suicide (e.g. weapons, toxic pharmaceuticals and pesticides). See Chapter 30.

Various types of policy regarding employment, leisure, planning of residential areas and availability of alcohol as well as legislation concerning health care and medical services and weapon ownership, are other typical examples of public health measures. Improvement of the work environment, especially for the health-care providers, and counteracting stress and burn-out that may lead to suicide are further public health strategies that are used in several countries.

Networks
National and international networks comprising researchers, professional and lay members are another category of population-oriented inputs. In Sweden, nationwide suicide prevention is co-ordinated by the National centre for suicide research and prevention of mental ill-health that follows up regional efforts. These regional efforts, which are adapted to local traditions and conditions, are implemented through regional networks that involve both professionals and lay people on a voluntary basis.

Research
In several countries, databases are being compiled[6] to permit monitoring and identification of trends and patterns of attempted and completed suicide, their sociodemographic and psychiatric characteristics as well as the kinds of treatment provided.

References

1. Support in Suicidal Crises. The Swedish national programme to develop suicide prevention. The National Council for Suicide Prevention, The National Board of Health and Welfare, The National Institute of Public Health, The National Centre for Suicide Research and Prevention of Mental Ill-health. Stockholm; 1995.

2. Jenkins R, Singh B. National suicide prevention strategies. *Psychiatr Fenn* 1999;**30**:9–30.

3. World Health Organization. Health-for-all targets. The health policy for Europe. Summary of the updated edition. Copenhagen: World Health Organization; 1992.

4. World Health Organization. Health 21: An introduction to the health for all policy framework for the WHO European region (European health for all series no. 5). 1998.

5. Preventing suicide: a resource series. Geneva: World Health Organization; 2000.
    1. A resource for general physicians.
    2. A resource for media professionals.
    3. A resource for teachers and other school staff.
    4. A resource for primary health care workers.
    5. A resource for prison officers.
    6. How to start a survivors' group.

6. Baxter D, Appleby L. Case register study of suicide risk in mental disorders. *Br J Psychiatry* 1999;**175**:322–326.

VIIA
Health-care perspectives

24

Examples of successful suicide prevention in psychiatry

Danuta Wasserman

Introduction

Suicide risk is particularly high among psychiatric patients shortly after discharge from hospital,[1,2] before they succeed in adjusting to their life situation and their relatives grasp that the safety net provided by the hospital has gone and has to be replaced. Life may feel empty and pointless. It may be difficult to take an interest in even the most ordinary activities. If there is no one holding the lifeline, suicide may ensue. The rate of mortality from suicide is elevated as early as 1 week after discharge, but elevated suicide risk remains for a whole year after discharge. The safety network represented by hospital falls away when patients are discharged, and it must be replaced by proper psychiatric rehabilitation activities and readjustment to life in the community. For lonely people with chronic mental illness, a home of one's own, secure finances, meaningful occupations to fill the days and human closeness are vitally important. Close co-operation between psychiatric services, social welfare authorities, voluntary organizations and family members is one of the preconditions for social rehabilitation and suicide prevention.

Suicide can be prevented

Adequate treatment of psychiatric patients and improved detection and treatment of psychiatric illnesses in the general population are essential strategies for suicide prevention. That the suicide-preventive effects of various types of psychiatric treatments have now been documented gives encouragement and hope.

Antidepressant drugs

Given that many patients who take their own lives are depressed and that

219

only a small minority receives adequate treatment for the depression, such treatment is a crucial part of suicide prevention. Depression may be treated in several ways, both with pharmacological and psychological methods. Unfortunately, controlled and randomized studies on sufficiently large numbers of suicidal patients are still lacking. What has been documented best to date is the effects of antidepressant drug treatments on the incidence of suicidal ideation, suicide attempts and completed suicide in *post hoc* meta-analyses of materials collected under a variety of conditions and for purposes other than evaluation of suicide prevention as such.

Montgomery et al.[3] performed meta-analyses of controlled, short-term efficacy studies of paroxetine compared with placebo effects in patients with moderate to severe major depression. Results show a significant reduction in suicidal thoughts among patient groups treated with antidepressants compared with the placebo group. The number of suicides per patient-year of exposure in the group receiving paroxetine was 5.6 times fewer than in the placebo group – albeit not at a statistically significant level – and the number of suicide attempts in the treatment group was half that in the placebo group. These results are in line with a previous meta-analysis performed by Beasley et al.[4], which showed that suicidal ideation decreased significantly in groups of patients treated with fluoxetine compared with placebo. The results of both these meta-analyses are consistent and particularly interesting, since Fawcett et al.[5] have shown that suicidal thoughts are a significant predictor of future suicide.

A naturalistic prospective follow-up study of people with affective disorders carried out by the US National Institute of Mental Health over several years showed a clear, although not statistically significant, reduction in suicidal behaviour among patients treated with fluoxetine.[6] Thus, the suspicion that this drug elevates suicide risk was not confirmed.

Suicide-preventive effects of treatment with older antidepressants have been studied at Zurich University Hospital.[7] Among patients treated for major depression with imipramine, there was a striking reduction in mortality from suicide in the group that had received long-term preventive treatment for recurrent depressions compared with groups that had not received preventive treatment (mortality rates of 5 per cent and 15 per cent, respectively).

Antidepressant drugs are a good tool, as long as psychiatrists learn how to use them. They should not be rejected on the grounds that they can be deliberately overdosed for the purpose of suicide. However, it should be borne in mind that treatment with antidepressants, even with the more modern selective serotonin reuptake inhibitors may give rise to some troublesome side effects. Antidepressants that activate serotonin-2 receptors in the central nervous system may induce anxiety and panic attacks at the beginning of the treatment. In the early phase of treatment, the severe anxiety usually persists while the depressed person ceases to suffer from psychomotor inhibition. If the patient's psychosocial problems remain and the suicidal person continues to find life hopeless and pointless, the result may be that certain patients take their own lives in this initial phase unless they are in close touch with doctors or other people who can hold the lifeline. The aim should therefore be to ensure that depressed, suicidal patients are invariably given combination treatment, with counselling or psychotherapy supplementing antidepressant drugs and vice versa.

Lithium

The efficacy of lithium treatment in preventing episodes of recurrent major affective illnesses mood disorder is well known. Long-term treatment with lithium has also proved to reduce suicide risk. Comparisons of suicide mortality for patients with unipolar and bipolar disorders receiving long-term lithium treatment compared with patients not receiving this treatment show that mortality due to suicide can be strikingly reduced in the group treated with lithium.[8–10]

The review by Tondo et al.[11] of several studies concerning large groups of patients with mood disorders shows clearly that long-term treatment with lithium reduces the risk of both suicide and attempted suicide. It has also been shown that discontinuing lithium treatment results in a risk of suicide and attempted suicide that is several times higher than the risk with continued treatment. Although these results are obtained from non-randomized controlled trials, they are consistent and suggest that careful and adequate lithium treatment of patients with unipolar and bipolar illness disorders helps to prevent suicidal acts. However, to reduce mortality from suicide, continuous treatment with lithium for a minimum of 2 years is required.[12]

Neuroleptics

Promising results, in terms of reduced suicide mortality, to only one-fifth of the expected rate for completed suicide in the population of schizophrenic patients have been reported when the suicide rate is adjusted for duration of treatment, in the case of treatment-resistant schizophrenics treated with clozapine.[13] A significant reduction in suicide was thus attained. A decreased number of the suicide attempts and a decrease in the suicide intent in neuroleptic-resistant patients with schizophrenia who were treated with clozapine have also been reported. Given that mortality from suicide is high among schizophrenic patients, these results, are very important. (See also Chapter 9.)

Psychotherapy

Cognitive behavioural psychotherapy for patients at high risk of repeated suicide attempts has proved to reduce this risk significantly up to several months after treatment is terminated.[14] Dialectical behavioural therapy also has documented effects in reducing repetition of suicide attempts for up to 1 year among female chronic suicide attempters with borderline personality disorder.[15] See Chapter 19.

Need for long-term treatment

Like pharmacological forms of treatment for suicidal patients, psychotherapy, especially for people with personality disorders, must be provided over a long period and, in some chronic cases, for several years.

The effects of treatment cannot be expected to persist when the short-term treatment ceases, since the suicidal patient's psychiatric, psychological and social background is often complex. Moreover, the suicidal process is a dynamic one. Problems may culminate again in a difficult life situation and intensification of the suicidal process may recur when a person's psychological ability to cope with difficulties in new circumstances deteriorates markedly. In the course of treatment, one should therefore teach patients to be prepared to seek help again if need be. Long-term or repeated preventive treatment is recommended at present only for the use of antidepressants for depressed patients, but such long-term treatments are also needed for psychotherapy.

Repetition of attempted suicide

Hawton et al.[16] scrutinized the results of several randomized controlled trials in which the effects on repetition of suicide attempts exerted by various psychosocial, psychotherapeutic and pharmacological treatments of patients who have deliberately harmed themselves had been studied. The results are promising, in terms of reduction of suicide-attempt repetition when problem-solving therapy was used. There was also a tendency for repetition of suicide attempts to decrease when emergency help was easily accessible by means of 'emergency contact cards', in contrast to standard after-care procedures.

A significant reduction in the number of repeat suicide attempts has also been obtained in the treatment of multiple repeaters with dialectical behaviour therapy compared with standard treatment, and in treatment with depot flupenthixol compared with placebo.

Evidence shows that repetition of self-destructive acts can be prevented, although it is still uncertain which treatments are the most effective. This is hardly surprising, since the treatment after a suicide attempt must be tailored individually, with psychiatric morbidity, personality traits and psychosocial situation of the suicidal person taken equally into account. There are several existing treatment options. However, there is also a need for new ones.

Psychosocial measures

Reduced repetition of suicide attempts

Motto et al.[17] reported a significantly lower mortality rate from suicide in a group of suicide-attempters who were followed up regularly, by correspondence, every month for the first 4 months after the suicide attempt, every second month for an additional 8 months, and every 3 months for an additional 4 years (i.e. a 5-year follow-up with 24 contacts) compared with a group who had not been followed up in this way.

Reduced suicidality among the elderly

The results of an intervention in Italy known as 'Tele-Help' and 'Tele-Check', which consists of a special telephone service for elderly people, are encouraging.[18] Tele-Help is an alarm system that permits active requests for help; Tele-Check is a systematic twice-weekly call from staff who check up on people's physical and mental state and provide emotional support. The results, which relate to more than 20,000 people aged 65 years and over who had access to this service 24 hours a day, showed that the service afforded social, medical and psychological support. Suicide mortality fell significantly, mental well-being was enhanced and hospital admissions and medical consultations decreased in number (see Chapter 22).

Lifelines

Analyses performed by Lester[19] at an aggregate level show a weak inverse association between the absolute number of suicide-prevention helping-hand services (such as Befrienders International, Samaritans and Lifelines) and the number of suicides that occur in the area covered by such services (see Chapter 22).

References

1. Appleby L, Shaw J, Amos T, et al. Suicide within 12 months of contact with mental health services: national clinical survey. *BMJ* 1999;**318:**1235–1239.

2. Goldacre M, Seagrott V, Hawton K. Suicide after discharge from psychiatric inpatient care. *Lancet* 1993;**342:**283–286.

3. Montgomery SA, Dunner DL, Dunbar GC. Reduction of suicidal thoughts with paroxetine in comparison with reference antidepressants and placebo. *Eur Neuropsychopharmacology* 1995; **5:**5–13.

4. Beasley CM, Dornseif BE, Bosomworth JC, et al. Fluoxetine and suicide: a meta-analysis of controlled trials of treatment for depression. *BMJ* 1991;**303:** 685–692.

5. Fawcett J, Scheftner WA, Fogg L, et al. Time-related predictors of suicide in major affective disorder. *Am J Psychiatry* 1990;**147:** 1189–1194.

6. Leon AC, Keller MB, Warshaw MG, et al. Prospective study of fluoxetine treatment and suicidal behavior in affectively ill subjects. *Am J Psychiatry* 1999;**156:** 195–201.

7. Angst J, Angst F, Stassen HH. Suicide risk in patients with major depressive disorder. J Clin Psychiatry 1999;**60(Suppl 2):**57–62.

8. Coppen A, Standish-Barry H, Bailey J. Long term lithium and mortality. *Lancet* 1990;**335:**1347.

9. Muller-Oerlinghausen B, Muser-Causemann B, Volk J. Suicides and parasuicides in a high-risk patient group on and off lithium long-term medication. *J Affect Disord* 1992;**25:**261–269.

10. Nilsson A. Lithium therapy and suicide risk. *J Clin Psychiatry* 1999;**60(Suppl 2):**85–88.

11. Tondo L, Jamison K, Baldessarini R. Effect of lithium maintenance on suicidal behavior in major mood disorders (Review). *Ann N Y Acad Sci* 1997;**836:**339–351.

12. Ahrens B, Muller-Oerlinghausen B, Graf F. Length of lithium treatment needed to eliminate the high mortality of affective disorders. *Br J Psychiatry* 1993;**163(Suppl 21):** 27–29.

13. Meltzer H. Suicide and schizophrenia: clozapine and the InterSePT study. International Clozaril/Leponex Suicide Prevention Trial. *J Clin Psychiatry* 1999;**60(Suppl 12):** 47–50.

14. Salkovskis P, Atha C, Storer D. Cognitive-behavioural problem solving in the treatment of patients who repeatedly attempt suicide, a controlled trial. *Br J Psychiatry* 1990;**157:**871–876.

15. Shearin EN, Linehan MM. Dialectical behaviour therapy for borderline personality disorder: theoretical and empirical foundations. *Acta Psychiatr Scand* 1994;**89(Suppl 379):** 61–68.

16. Hawton K, Arensman E, Townsend E, et al. Deliberate self-harm: systematic review of efficacy of psychosocial and pharmacological treatments in preventing repetition. *BMJ* 1998;**317:**441–447.

17. Motto J, Heilbron D, Juster R, Bostrom A. Communication as a suicide prevention programme. In: Soubrier JP, Vedrinne J (eds). Depression et suicide. Paris: Pergamon Press; 1981:148–154.

18. De Leo D, Carollo G, Dello Buono M. Lower suicide rates associated with a Tele-Help/Tele-Check service for the elderly at home. *Am J Psychiatry* 1995;**152:**632–634.

19. Lester D. The effectiveness of suicide prevention centers. *Suicide Life Threat Behav* 1993;**23:**263–267.

25

An example of a suicide-preventive strategy: general practitioners' training

Wolfgang Rutz

The Gotland study

Detecting and treating depressive conditions as the principal feature of the suicidal process was the aim of the Gotland study. This study was implemented as a training programme in the early 1980s, evaluated until the early 1990s and followed up with maintenance training until 1998. The study, with its success and shortcomings, illustrates the potential but also the limitations of medical and psychiatric services – in terms of how well they treat and monitor psychiatric morbidity, the immediate cause of most suicides – in fulfilling their obligatory duties.

The Swedish island of Gotland, with a population of some 60,000, is a psychiatric 'sector' and also an epidemiologically 'transparent' laboratory. Despite their apparently high quality of life and the beautiful surroundings, the inhabitants of Gotland have undergone dramatic social transition. In the 1970s, the island was one of the 'black spots' for suicidality in Sweden: its suicide rate was among the highest in Sweden, well above urban rates. One feature was the high and, very often, violent suicidality, often in females. The prescription rate in Gotland for antidepressants, the lowest in Sweden, was offset by high over-prescription of sedative, anxiolytic and hypnotic drugs.

In this alarming situation, initiatives for a training campaign were taken by general practitioners (GPs), who were eager to help their patients but felt helpless and incompetent. To help the GPs to tackle the island's depression and suicide problems, the local psychiatric department and the Swedish Committee for Prevention and Treatment of Depressions (the PTD Committee) jointly initiated a training programme on depression in primary health care. This comprehensive, structured programme comprised two courses of 2 days each and was offered, over a 2-year period, to all the GPs in Gotland. It covered most aspects of detection and monitoring of depressive disorders, and all but one GP participated. The

225

programme was given in a somewhat luxurious hotel environment deemed conducive to learning. The two consecutive days and night in between afforded time and scope for interaction, discussion and sharing of personal clinical and private experience, as well as lectures, video presentations and case discussions. The participants were able to influence the programme after the first year by pointing out what it lacked, and they were given all the teaching material in written form, for use in training their own teams.

The problem of depression and its detection and monitoring was presented in an integrative and synoptic way. The process of becoming depressed and suicidal, and also the process of recovering, were described as multifactorial. Accordingly, multidisciplinary and multimodal intervention and help were said to be required. The sometimes crucial and inevitable need for psychopharmacological treatment was explained, as was the need for psychotherapeutic follow-up and support in a process-related way. Psychotherapy and pharmacotherapy were presented as complementary approaches rather than as alternative strategies, according to the maxim that 'there is a time for everything'.

The distinction between 'endogenous' and 'exogenous' aetiology was consequently avoided, as were contradictions between the psychodynamic, psychosocial and biological approaches. Instead, a stress-vulnerability model was used. The need for integrative thinking was therefore emphasized in terms of multifactoriality and the need for process-related action. This 'holistic' approach also resulted in efforts to describe depression not as a distinct nosological entity associated with various comorbidities but, rather, as a state connected with anxiety, drug abuse, alcoholism and temporary personality changes. Various types of destructive behaviour were also examined as symptoms that are often related to and caused by depression.

With its structured and holistic presentation, the training was highly appreciated and brought about a significant improvement in GPs' capacity to diagnose, treat and monitor depressive conditions. During the 3 years after the training programme – the period of its maximum impact – a wide range of interrelated results connected with the training were observed. Referrals for depression to the local psychiatric institution and also the number of days of sick leave for depressive and apathetic conditions fell by more than 50 per cent in Gotland. The amount of in-patient care at the local psychiatric clinic for depressive conditions dropped by 70 per cent and suicides decreased by some two-thirds. Prescription of antidepressants rose from less then 50 per cent of the Swedish average to over 80 per cent; conversely, there was a decrease of 30 per cent in the number of sedatives, anxiolytics and hypnotics prescribed, in relation to the Swedish average, normalizing the previous over-prescription. Three years after the training, thanks to improved diagnosis of recurrent depressive conditions, lithium prescription also rose by 30 per cent.

Another recent finding is that the seasonality of suicide patterns in Gotland, which was fairly marked in the 1980s, decreased significantly during the 1990s. It may confirm that the basic problem in Gotland before the training project was one of underdiagnosis and undertreatment of seasonal depression, resulting in a high number of depression-related suicides. This situation was improved by the training inputs.[1]

The need for continuous training

However, these changes were only temporary. By the end of the decade the suicide numbers had returned to their baseline values or slightly above, and the need for continued and updating training was apparent. New courses began in the early 1990s and follow-up refresher courses were provided at intervals of about 2 years until 1998.

A special cost–benefit calculation showed that the training programme, which cost roughly SEK 400,000, resulted in substantial savings for society during the 3-year period of its maximum impact owing to the reductions in morbidity, suicide mortality, in-patient care and spending on drugs.[2]

Male suicidality unchanged

Detailed scrutiny of the suicide-preventive effects of this training programme revealed that the positive change of reduced suicidality was found mainly in the group of female suicides, while male suicides were unaffected.[3] The male suicides were mostly violent. Moreover, unlike the relatively few women in Gotland who committed suicide in the 1990s, and who were mostly known to the health-care services, the great majority of men who committed suicide were known only to the police, tax authorities or social welfare authorities that deal with alcoholics.

The training, focused as it was on improving the quality of GPs' recognition and monitoring of depression, evidently had no positive impact on male suicidality in Gotland, since the men concerned committed suicide without coming into contact with health-care services. In the few cases when such contact existed, the men were diagnosed as having personality disorders, showing sociopathic behaviour or being drug abusers, and were often considered untreatable owing to their uncooperative behaviour, 'psychopathic' acting-out, aggression or lack of compliance with and motivation for treatment. Research shows that depressive and suicidal men usually display atypical depressive symptoms. If they casually ask for help, their depression is often neither recognized nor effectively treated.

In view of the persistently high male suicide rate, the follow-up training

programmes placed heavier emphasis on depressive symptoms and suicidal behaviour in males. A scale that focuses on the typical 'atypical'
male depressive symptoms was developed, presenting the typical features of male depression: impaired stress tolerance, acting-out, aggression, low impulse control, irritability, indecision, abuse tendencies,
temporarily 'antisocial' behaviour and inheritance of tendencies towards
suicide, depression and substance abuse. This scale was based on clinical experience and has now been tested for several years as a screening
instrument to detect depression in males who are in contact with primary
care or other health-care or social services. The scale is currently being
subjected to scientific evaluation and validation. Since this 'Gotland Male
Depression Scale' has been taught as a screening instrument to local primary health-care staff and presented in the Gotland mass media, a
decrease in male suicides on Gotland has also been observed.

At present, the concept of male depression and suicidality is increasingly the focus of scientific interest and is being mentioned in a growing
number of contexts. However, since most of the male depressives who
commit suicide are not in contact with any health-care services,
approaches must be developed to reach them by involving other players
in society – the men's workplaces, trade unions, social networks, families
and friends, as well as the mass media.[4]

International experience

Training aimed at better recognition and monitoring of depressive and
depression-related conditions in primary care appears to prevent suicide. Data show the importance of GPs as the front line in diagnosis and
treatment of depression. Even if one controlled study in a setting much
differing from the Gotland situation failed to replicate the positive outcome of the Gotland study as a whole,[5,6] experience from training programmes in Switzerland, the UK, Ireland, Hungary, the Baltic states, the
USA, Canada and elsewhere indicates that training results in increased
specific treatment of depression, with antidepressants and lithium being
prescribed more and non-specific sedatives, hypnotics and anxiolytics
less. This may be expected to have a suicide-preventive effect.[1,7–10]

Case history

The patient was a journalist, 52 years old, also known as an artist and
writer: an intellectual, opinion moulder, entertainer and presenter of a
popular television programme. He came from an adventurous family of
artists and writers. His father had been a creative teacher and heavy
drinker, with long unproductive periods. Divorced many years previously,

the patient was now involved with a younger woman. The relationship was functioning relatively smoothly, and the couple had one child. He was in full swing, with high public visibility, and intensely active in a wide-ranging social network.

For 6 months, he had been feeling increasingly uneasy, especially in the mornings. He was experiencing growing restlessness, a sense of hopelessness and a feeling of being a fake. He had difficulty in making even minor, everyday decisions. He felt overwhelmed by everyday problems, paralysed – but, at the same time, he remained active in his work. He was talkative and sociable, but his concentration and real interest in social life were now habitually lacking.

His sleep was increasingly fragmented. Especially at night, he frequently experienced an almost irresistible, compulsive urge to take his own life, and he was becoming ever more frightened of being unable to resist this urge. He had made several nocturnal excursions to remote places with concrete plans to commit suicide by hanging, jumping or asphyxiation in his car. He reported an inner struggle on these occasions, after which he finally managed to return home. Shocked by this experience, he had sought psychiatric help following his own research in preparation for a programme on male helplessness.

He made a pleasant, talkative, professional, easy-going and social adequate impression. No inhibition was evident. He reported increasing consumption of alcohol – mostly wine – to 'calm down'. He stated that he was no longer able to write, since he lacked new ideas, but could manage his programme on a 'routine' basis. He had received no reactions from others – nobody had noticed his problems – but he told of his deepening despair and was horrified at his own compulsive suicidal urges.

The diagnosis was male depression, with acute suicidality. The recommended treatment was selective serotonin reuptake inhibitors (SSRI) combined with weekly individual psychotherapy sessions focusing on acceptance of his limitations, helplessness, weakness and inability to cope with every demand, plus family-therapy sessions with his family to monitor his suicidality. Recovery took 8 weeks, and the patient is currently receiving long-term maintenance treatment with supportive and clarifying psychotherapy and psychopharmacology.

References

1. Rihmer Z, Rutz W, Pihlgren H. Decreasing tendency of seasonality in suicide may indicate lowering rate of depressive suicides in the population. *Psychiatry Res* 1998;**16:**233–240.

2. Rutz W. Evaluation of an educational programme on depressive disorders given to general practitioners in Gotland. Short- and long-term effects. Dissertation. Sweden: Linköping University; 1992:1–116.

3. Rutz W, von Knorring L, Pihlgren H, Rihmer Z, Wålinder J. Prevention of male suicides: lessons from the Gotland study. *Lancet* 1995;**345:**524.

4. Rutz W. Improvement of care for people suffering from depression: the need for comprehensive education. *Int Clin Psychopharmacol* 1999;**14(Suppl 3):**27–33.

5. Thomson C, Stevens L, Ostler K. The Hampshire Depression Project: a methodology for assessing the value of general practice education for depression. *Int J Meth Psychiat Res* 1996;**6:**527–531.

6. Thompson C, Kinmoth AL, Stevens L et al. Effects of a clinical-practice guideline and practice-based education on detection and outcome of depression in primary care: Hampshire Depression Project randomised controlled trial. *Lancet* 2000; **355:**185–191.

7. McKeon P, Garigan P, Slobhan C. Aware of depression. *Ir Med J* 1989;**82:**2–3.

8. Michel K, Valach L. Suicide prevention: spreading the Gospel to general practitioners. *Br J Psychiatry* 1992;**160:**757–760.

9. Standart SH, Drinkwater C, Scott J. Multidisciplinary training in the detection, assessment and management of depressions in primary care. *Prim Care Psychiatry* 1997;**3:**89–93.

10. Bodlund O. Most depressed patients can be treated in primary care. *Läkartidningen* 2000;**97:**1244–9.

26

Collaboration between psychiatrists and other physicians

Jean-Pierre Soubrier

Suicide in different medical settings

It is well known that up to 60 per cent of suicidal people, and in some studies even more, have consulted one or more physicians just 1–2 months before their suicidal act, whether its outcome was temporary (for attempters) or final (for those who died).[1,2] As patients, these people usually come into contact with general practitioners or specialists in various fields of somatic medicine. The setting may be a private surgery or a public out-patient clinic, and besides general practice the main specialities of the doctors concerned are internal medicine (with its various subdivisions – cardiology, gastroenterology, endocrinology and so on), orthopaedics, neurology, gynaecology, otorhinolaryngology and urology. The presuicidal phase is of the utmost importance in prevention, and medical staff who meet patients in this category therefore bear a heavy burden of responsibility.[3]

General practitioners, and to a lesser extent other physicians, are frequently the first and sometimes the only professional players in the drama of suicide. What can they do, and what should they refrain from doing? What kind of help is needed? For anyone who is not a trained psychiatrist, dealing with suicidal patients is a difficult task. Psychiatrists may play a vital role in their care and treatment. However, no one should work unaided with suicidal patients and in suicide prevention. Teamwork in which a psychiatrist plays a key role may be a solution.

Suicide-prevention team

Every medical setting should include structures and routines whereby a psychiatrist instructs the staff concerned in how to deal with suicidal patients and their families, and also in suicide prevention. Preventing suicide is a burdensome task, and it is therefore advisable for such work to be carried out by a suicide-prevention team of several people. A psychiatrist should head the team, which should include professionals from various fields, such as a psychologist, a social worker and a psychiatric nurse. The team's close collaboration is a prerequisite for its success.

The suicide-prevention team may be the source of knowledge and be in charge of current training both in the psychiatric clinic and in the whole hospital. It may also serve as a link between health-care services and the relevant authorities in the community. Another function of the team may be to ensure continuous application of modern treatment and preventive methods within existing routines. A quality-assurance programme could be established, and this means that quality indicators need to be defined. Examples of such indicators are the percentage of suicide-attempt patients examined by a psychiatrist within 24 hours of their attempt and suicidal patients' average wait to see a psychiatrist after referral.

Training may be provided on a regular basis to general practitioners and other doctors.[1,4,5] Topics should include:

- reasons why suicidal people consult somatic doctors;
- when suicidal patients should be referred to a psychiatrist or admitted to hospital;
- how to communicate with suicidal patients' relatives; and
- the need for follow-up after a suicide attempt.

Other important team duties include offering support to staff in emergency departments and intensive care units and drawing up rules of conduct for the aftermath of a suicide on the ward.

Co-operation with somatic physicians

Liaison between psychiatrists, general practitioners and other medical practitioners who treat suicidal patients has a profound impact on the course of the suicidal process at all stages. This impact is not always as positive as might be expected. A certain taboo remains, reinforced by supposed ethical considerations and respect for privacy. This may be one explanation why suicide figures are underestimates and suicide prevention is fairly difficult to implement.

Very often, suicidal patients approach the non-psychiatric physician with somatic complaints of one kind or another, and cite several examples of different symptoms without expressing any overt suicidal communication during their visit. Either these patients do not associate their suicidal tendencies with somatic symptoms, or they consider suicidal ideation a sign of weakness and are often ashamed of their suicidal thoughts or plans to take their own life. They mention their feelings of helplessness and worthlessness and their fears only in vague terms. The emotional instability and low self-esteem so characteristic of suicidal people may, instead, be compensated for by an impression of strength and competence. There is thus a marked discrepancy between patients' underlying desperation and what they express verbally during the consultation. Physicians expect suicidal patients to be depressed and may therefore miss suicidality unless they penetrate more deeply into the diagnosis. Symptoms of depression may be masked by physical symptoms and pain, accompanied by sleep disorders, fatigue, irritability and anxiety.[2]

For the above reasons, it is hardly surprising if initial and also subsequent contacts between somatic doctors or general practitioners and their suicidal patients fail to prevent suicidal acts. Psychotic and alcohol or other substance abusers may present relatively surmountable problems of suicide-risk assessment. If they are promptly referred to appropriate specialists who are better trained to treat such patients, their suicidal acts may be averted.

Clearly, other physicians and general practitioners should also be trained in the careful evaluation of all patients who may be suspected of somatization or who may have psychosomatic symptoms. Clinical intuition, experience and common sense are major tools in this context, but they must be supplemented by education and training in basic suicidal assessment.[6,7]

Patient–physician relationship

All doctors should be trained in communicating with suicidal patients, to optimize diagnosis and treatment. Communication between suicidal patients and their physicians is positively or negatively affected by the physician's attitudes towards the suicide and his or her degree of communication skill and psychological preparedness to deal with self-destructive behaviour. Suicidal patients' expectations of and attitudes towards their physicians also profoundly influence the communication and compliance with treatment recommendations.

Referral for psychiatric evaluation

Whenever there is the slightest suspicion of suicidality, patients must be referred to a psychiatrist or psychologist. Such referrals must also take place when patients present with mental disorders, fail to take antidepressant medication or to comply with other treatment, or express a desire for psychological help. Patients must also be referred when they have a personal or family history of attempted suicide and lack social support.

However, seeing a psychiatrist is the dominant fear of many suicidal patients, who are apprehensive that such contact may in some way confirm relatives' opinion that they are of unsound mind. A written referral and active, urgent follow-up are therefore imperative.

A simple suggestion to a person to approach a psychiatrist can be directly counterproductive. Before referring patients one should inform them and, if possible, their relatives that specialist help is necessary. The referral should not be perceived by the patient as abandonment; instead, it should be a joint decision. It is helpful in this context to explain the beneficial effects of various forms of psychotherapy and drugs. The primary care or other physician should also ensure follow-up of the contact with the psychiatrist to whom the patient is referred. This is because of the need to know whether the patient has approached the psychiatrist or not. A precondition for successful referral is for the referring doctor to have well-established contacts and to be personally acquainted with private psychiatrists or public out-patient and in-patient psychiatric departments. This is all the more important if the patient is isolated and lacks social support and protective factors.

When to hospitalize a suicidal patient

In some cases, immediate hospitalization is appropriate.[3] This applies to patients with recurrent severe thoughts of suicide, serious intent to die, major depression with anxiety and agitation or psychoses such as schizophrenia and manic–depressive disorder. It also applies to patients with borderline personalities in traumatic life situations. Admission is further required when a suicidal patient has poor family or social support. However, evaluation is no easy matter when no obvious signs of profound or severe mental disorder are present.

Emergency admission and admission to an intensive care unit

Collaboration between psychiatrists and the staff of intensive care units and emergency departments is essential for patients who have survived a suicide attempt. Confronting suicidal patients is often traumatic for all medical staff in the units concerned. Hospital staff are all too seldom trained to deal with and understand complex psychological problems. The suicidal patient constitutes a threat to staff's professional role – that of saving lives – and also evokes their own anxiety about death and threatens their personal integrity. Staff reactions are variable, and include uncertainty, fear, anxiety, uneasiness and guilt. These feelings may result in distancing, escape reactions, irritation and aggression, but also in interest and empathy. In general, medical staff are often dissatisfied with the amount of help they can give patients and their relatives, owing to the lack of knowledge and shortage of time, and also to poor collaboration with psychiatrists.[8]

Contact with relatives

The psychiatrist's most important and usual role in the emergency setting is to establish contact with the suicidal patient's relatives. It is well known that people who have attempted suicide belong to one of the major risk groups for completed suicide. Family members are often under psychological duress and need advice, psychological support and sometimes psychiatric treatment. Last but not least, psychiatrists may help physicians to comfort relatives or close friends of patients who have died from suicide. Programmes for surviving relatives must be encouraged. (See also Chapter 28.)

Follow-up and treatment planning

The psychiatrist's task is to intervene in the suicidal process and to slow it. This can be achieved only by ensuring follow-up, with psychosocial, psychological and medical care, with or without medication. Eventually, some patients may be referred to their general practitioner for follow-up and treatment. The general practitioner must then be in a position to plan treatment in co-operation with the patients and their families, and have easy access to a psychiatrist or suicide-prevention team for consultation whenever necessary, and to discuss cases during the follow-up period. To enhance the support they can provide, general practitioners need regular training programmes.[1,9]

Suicide on the ward

A dramatic situation like suicide in a hospital may induce typical post-traumatic stress syndrome among staff. In such situations a suicide-prevention team should perform a therapeutic function by debriefing the staff and commenting on the clinical aspects of the case. In this process, co-operation with forensic physicians and forensic psychiatrists may be necessary, within a postvention programme (see also Chapter 27).

Continuous training

Collaboration between psychiatrists, psychologists, general practitioners and other doctors should be extensive, owing to its importance in the treatment of suicidal patients and in relieving psychological tensions that may be experienced by staff.[5] Good co-operation and continuous training of physicians in primary care and other fields by their psychiatrist colleagues and the suicide-prevention team are essential elements in successful suicide prevention at every stage.

The suicide-prevention team should play a key role not only in skills development but also in terms of emotional debriefing.

References

1. Rutz W, von Knorring L, Wallinder J. Long term effects of an education programme for general practitioners given by the Swedish committee for the prevention and treatment of depression. *Acta Psychiatr Scand* 1992;**85:**83–88.

2. Wolk-Wasserman D. Contacts of suicidal neurotic and prepsychotic/psychotic patients and their significant others with public care institutions before the suicide attempt. *Acta Psychiatr Scand* 1987;**75:**358–372.

3. Litman R. Hospital suicides: lawsuits and standards. *Suicide Life Threat Behav* 1982;**12:**212–220.

4. Soubrier JP, Debout M, Bertolote JM, et al. Guide de l'entretien avec un patient suicidaire. Paris: Lundbeck-France; 1998.

5. World Health Organization. Preventing suicide: a resource for general physicians. Mental behavioural disorders. Department of Mental Health, Social Change and Mental Health. Geneva. 2000.

6. Beck AT, Brown GK, Steer RA. Suicide ideation at its worst point: a prediction of eventual suicide in psychiatric outpatients. *Suicide Life Threat Behav* 1999;**29:**1–4.

7. Jacobs DG. Guide to suicide assessment and intervention. San Francisco: Jossey Bass Publishers; 1999.

8. Wolk-Wasserman D. The intensive care unit and the suicide attempt patient. *Acta Psychiatr Scand* 1985;**71:**581–595.

9. Soubrier JP. Definitions du suicide. Signification de la prévention. *Ann Medicopsychol* 1999; **157:**526–529.

27
The work environment for health-care staff

Danuta Wasserman

Vulnerability of psychiatric staff

There are reports that show that the incidence of suicidal acts is particularly high among health professionals. The fact that health-care workers are constantly confronted with issues of life and death, and with suicidal patients, raises questions relating to the work environment for psychiatric care providers and the need for regular training, supervision and support.[1,2]

At every psychiatric clinic or department, there should be routines that allow scope for raising issues of failure and inadequacy in connection with treatment of suicidal patients and a patient's suicide. The purpose is to help staff cope with their own emotional experience, take a stand on personal existential issues and develop professionally.

Attempted suicide and suicide runs directly counter not only to the instinct of self-preservation, but also to the role of health-care staff as those who provide health care and save lives. This is why it is not unusual for people close to suicide (who violate this role) to be given a negative reception. These negative feelings may sometimes be very strong among the staff.[3]

Sound routines keep chaos and anxiety in check

Powerful emotional reactions in the form of indifference, rejection and antipathy should be explored fully, since they have a profound influence on suicidal patients and may even promote suicide. Constant awareness of the nocebo effect (i.e. the harmful impact on patients of therapists' conduct, procedure and treatment) is necessary. Failing to admit compulsorily a patient who is at high risk of suicide and opting for a less active treatment instead or omitting to treat a patient with antidepressants may be expressions of negative reactions on the staff's part, rather than of their concern for the patient.[3,4]

Negative countertransference reactions may arise even in the best-trained personnel. The suicidal conflict is, fundamentally, a highly aggressive one and it is hardly surprising that it affects staff. Bearing in mind that the behaviour of the staff may provoke or contribute to suicide should be as self-evident as awareness of the beneficial effects (placebo effects) of a trustful contact between patient and physician, especially since the reaction of the staff can have a nocebo effect and lead to the patient's suicide.

Every department in which work with suicidal persons is performed should have documented routines for diagnosis and treatment to ensure that appropriate action is taken. Good routines are particularly important in treatment of suicidal people since ways of working with suicidal patients are strongly influenced by staff's attitudes, their state of mental health and well-being and their outlook on life, including values regarding various ethical and moral issues.

Routines and documentation relieve staff's anxiety and uncomfortable emotions, and also promote good care, commitment and the creativity that is released when chaos is kept in check. Conversely, unhealthy work conditions may result in 'burn-out', with apathetic, irritable or dismissive attitudes towards patients.[5-9]

Dealing with a suicidal person is arduous work, and an ability to hold the lifeline makes high demands in terms of knowledge and personal characteristics. Staff who work with suicidal people therefore need regular training and support, and also supervision in their day-to-day work.

Case history:
A patient's suicide – an unbearable experience

Hans, aged 30 years, a hospital ward nurse and the only child of two elderly doctors, was admitted to a psychiatric ward after a 2-week stay in the intensive care unit after throwing himself in front of an underground train. He was beset by problems. On the relationship front, his fiancée had broken off their engagement shortly before the wedding was due to take place; at work, major reorganizations were taking place and he was facing a demotion. His real wish was to be a doctor, but his school grades were not good enough.

The staff at the psychiatric ward thought that they had come to know Hans fairly well, and after a few weeks' care he was granted his first weekend leave. Before his departure, a doctor met him briefly. Hans appeared calm and the doctor had little time on that particular day to explore in depth his state of mind or how prepared he was for an encounter with the real-life world outside the hospital. Nor had his relatives been contacted; Hans' statement that he was going to spend the weekend with his elderly parents was simply taken on trust.

On the Monday, all the staff were shocked to receive a request to identify the body of one of their patients, brought to the hospital during the weekend. It was Hans, who had lain down on the underground track late in the evening on the same day he had left the hospital. There, invisible in the darkness, he had been run over and killed.

It was a dreadful experience for everyone on the ward. This applied not least to the doctor who had last met and talked to Hans before his leave. Even several years later, this doctor related that the event had had such a tremendous impact on him that still, every time he was reminded of it, he became agitated and his heart began to pound rapidly.

Support for staff after a suicidal act of the patient

Immediate routine measures

After a suicide or suicide attempt has taken place, the questions of how to inform the patient's relatives, who should do so, and how to protect and inform the other patients must be settled without delay. The person in charge of the ward must also decide which tasks should be cancelled for the rest of the day in order to give the personnel time for meetings and emotional working-through.

Information must also be given to the administrative head of the institution as well as to the police or other authorities. This procedure varies from country to country and is regulated by national laws.

Contacts with relatives

Relatives should be informed, without delay, face to face in their own home or asked to come to the hospital. Giving them the news by telephone is inappropriate. It is important to give relatives a chance of meeting the staff members who looked after the patient before the suicide, and also to facilitate the access to therapy if they wish.

Immediate emotional support for staff

Being a member of the medical staff means facing suffering and death on a daily basis, and every so often encountering emotionally trying situations. But a patient's suicide is among the most daunting experiences a psychiatrist and members of the psychiatric staff can undergo. It is therefore extremely important to be able to work through the feelings that are aroused.[10]

A suicidal act is a tragedy that affects the whole staff team and the entire clinic or department. Not only strong feelings but also irrational explanations, projections of guilt on to others and self-reproaches are brought up. An immediate opportunity for working through the traumatic emotional aftermath of a suicidal act, individually and in a group, must be given to all the staff, as must the opportunity for everyone to relate the event from his or her own point of view. It is important for those affected to be able to speak freely of their feelings and express their anger, sorrow and despair.

All the health-care staff involved should take part in such meeting. The people who are affected most deeply often wish to withdraw, and take sick leave or holiday. Sometimes one meeting is not enough and additional meetings may be necessary. Staff who react very strongly should be given the opportunity for individual therapy. It is also vital for the person who chairs such a discussion to have a structure – one that does not, however, stifle the personal emotional reactions that arise during the meeting. This discussion of the staff's emotions should be led by someone who was not involved in the event and, preferably, is employed elsewhere. Conflicts between coworkers may come to the fore in this kind of situation, but it is important for these to be dealt with in some other context. The first impressions from the initial meeting must always be summarized by the person who heads the group.

Developing knowledge after the suicidal event

Within some 4–6 weeks after a suicide has taken place in the ward or department, a 'psychological autopsy' can be carried out. This method was developed at the Suicide Prevention Center in Los Angeles in the 1950s.[11] The purpose of such a review is to improve all the staff's skills by reconstructing the suicidal process up to the time of the suicidal act, and to go through the whole treatment process systematically. Strong emotional reactions may also arise in this kind of retrospective review. It provides a good opportunity for these reactions to be heard and support to be provided for those in need. A new assessment of diagnostics and treatment options should be carried out with the aim of integrating the staff's newly acquired knowledge with their previous knowledge and experience. The material from the autopsy and the police investigation can also be used. The entire review and the final assessment should be entered in the patient's medical records.

In many clinics, a retrospective review after a suicide attempt has taken place in the in-patient or out-patient department has been introduced as a routine since the staff is usually very highly motivated to reassess the actions taken in the treatment.

Training and supervision

A plan for a clinic offering regular training in suicidology – diagnostics, treatment and preventive strategies – can be a helpful measure. Moreover, individual supervision of staff should be available. Supervision develops not only the staff's knowledge of psychiatry, but also their psychotherapeutic skills and contributes to the emotional maturity. Individual support is particularly important for psychiatrists who are responsible for supervising other staff groups in their own departments, somatic doctors at adjacent clinics, and general practitioners.[1]

Enhancing the quality of suicide-preventive work

Wherever staff work with suicidal patients, there should be:

- a plan for training courses for all the staff;
- an individual plan for supervision of each staff member;
- an action programme to be implemented when a suicide or suicide attempt takes place on the ward;
- simple monitoring of suicide attempts and suicides.

More advanced registration of all suicidal acts that have taken place at the clinic or outpatient department can include diagnostic and treatment data, and also information on waiting times and the duration of treatment, in order to provide basic and specific local knowledge of the efficacy of treatment methods used.

References

1. Ramberg IL, Wasserman D. Working conditions in psychiatric care of suicidal patients in Sweden. In press.

2. Samuelsson M, Gustavsson JP, Pettersson IL, Arnetz B, Åsberg M. Suicidal feelings and work environment in psychiatric nursing personnel. *Soc Psychiatry Epidemiol* 1997;**32:**391–397.

3. Wolk-Wasserman D. Some problems connected with the treatment of suicide attempt patients: transference and countertransference aspects. *Crisis* 1987;**8:**69–82.

4. Deary IJ, Agius RM, Sadler A. Personality and stress in consultant psychiatrists. *Int J Soc Psychiatry* 1996;**42:**112–123.

5. Oberlander LB. Work satisfaction among community-based mental health service providers: the association between work environment and work satisfaction. *Community Ment Health J* 1990;**26:**517–532.

6. Pettersson IL, Arnetz BB, Arnetz JE, Hörte LG. Work environment, skills utilization and health of Swedish nurses: results from a National Questionnaire Study. *Psychother Psychosom* 1995;**64:**20–31.

7. Schulz R, Greenley JR, Brown R. Organization, management and client effects on staff burnout. *J Health Soc Behav* 1995;**36:**333–345.

8. Shinn M, Rosario M, Morch H, Chestnut DE. Coping with job stress and burnout in the human services. *J Pers Soc Psychol* 1984;**46:**864–876.

9. Thomsen S, Dallender, J, Soares, J, Nolan P, Arnetz B. Predictors of

a healthy workplace for Swedish and English psychiatrists. *Br J Psychiatry* 1998;**173:**80–84.

10. Beskow J, Runeson B, Åsgård U. Ethical aspects of psychological autopsy. *Acta Psychiatr Scand* 1991;**84:**482–487.

11. Shneidman E. The psychological autopsy. *Suicide Life Threat Behav* 1981;**11:**325–340.

28

Family involvement in suicide prevention and postvention: a psychoeducational perspective

Karen Dunne-Maxim and Edward J Dunne

The wise clinician

'A suicidal depression is a kind of spiritual winter, frozen, sterile, unmoving.' These are the words of A Alvarez, whose poignant memoir *A savage God: a study of suicide* [1] describes his relationship with the poet Sylvia Plath, who died by suicide, and his own near-fatal suicide attempt by taking sleeping pills. Not all people who contemplate suicide seek help during their crisis. However, when they do, it can raise extreme anxiety in the treating clinician, who often feels helpless in the face of such profound despair. The suicidal patient plunges the clinician into a life and death struggle, challenging him or her to use all his or her resources to preserve and strengthen the patient's will to live. A death by suicide is permanent; the clinician often sees it as preventable.

The wise clinician who wishes to approach the suicidal person marshaling all possible resources should include the family as part of the patient's treatment team from the beginning. For instance, in order to assess the patient's home environment adequately for safety, it is important to know if there are lethal weapons that are accessible to the patient. Information about this needs to be corroborated by the patient's family. Suicidal patients frequently minimize their danger and exaggerate the availability of help as a way of avoiding hospitalization. The clinician needs to make an independent assessment of these variables, by a thorough investigation of the circumstances with the family.

Patients do better when families are involved

Involving the family in the treatment of psychiatric illnesses is a relatively new phenomenon, but in the USA it has become the usual practice for treating patients with varied medical conditions. Most treatment centers operate support groups for families of their patients with cancer or heart disease. Families are increasingly attending seminars to learn more about their loved one's illness, how to assist with medication compliance, monitor progress and even assist with medication administration. The effort to create a collaborative team of physician, patient and family has even undermined the traditional conspiracy between the physician and patient in keeping the secret of a terminal prognosis from the family. Family involvement in medical treatment is common in the USA because patients generally do better with it.

The field of psychiatric treatment has been a late bloomer in this movement, but as clinicians recognize the success of family involvement in physical medicine it has begun to take root. The new psychiatric treatments have had to struggle against a long tradition of viewing the family as the cause of many mental illnesses and the attempt to extrude the patient from the family as a means of a cure.

For their part, patients themselves may have contributed to the exclusion of families from psychiatric treatment because of the stigma associated with mental illnesses and suicide. This is not unlike the situation for cancer victims 40 years ago, who were so ashamed of the diagnosis that they chose to die rather than seek treatment. Today many people kill themselves rather than accept the stigma associated with getting treatment for a 'mental' illness. Some families are still reluctant to admit that their relative is mentally ill. Fortunately, this is changing, owing to efforts of major advocacy groups for the mentally ill as well as increased public awareness. Many patients, however, still do not want to involve their families in their treatment because of their sense of shame. They believe they should be able to pull themselves out of it on their own. It becomes the task of the clinician to convince the patient to co-operate with this new plan. Generally, the result of openly discussing the suicidal thoughts and feelings with family members provides reason to believe that help may be only a spoken word away. Suddenly, suicidal ideation is no longer a sin to be hidden; it is a problem to be solved.[2]

Reasons for involving the family

Additional information

Families may provide additional information on the patient's behavior. This is especially true with anger and impulsivity, since the individual patient is less likely to report these symptoms. In a case from our clinic, a clinician was treating a 26-year-old man for depression as an out-patient. After a discussion with the patient's wife, however, who reported on the client's angry outbursts and impulsivity (a red flag in assessing lethality of suicidal intent) and cited one evening when, in a rage, her husband threw their fish tank against the wall, killing their prize collection of tropical fish, the treatment plan shifted dramatically to have a new focus on safety and suicide prevention.

Influencing attitudes

Educating the family about the nuances of the illness can affect their attitudes and behavior toward the patient. It has also been shown that educating patients and families about the illness is an effective means of decreasing hospitalizations, reducing length of stay and lowering the rate of suicide among people with major mental illnesses such as schizophrenia and bipolar disorders.[3] It has also been argued[4] that the high prevalence of major mental illnesses among suicidal people strongly recommends this psychoeducational approach.

In one instance, a young professional woman whose husband was deeply depressed stated that she realizes how counterproductive her interactions with her husband had been. She remembers nagging him about household chores. 'I thought he was being lazy. Now I realize that all his energy was devoted to staying alive.' When she learned more about the illness she was able to change her nagging stance to a more collaborative one. As his depression lifted with the aid of psychotherapy and medication, she was able to relish in his recovery.

Providing a resource

Assessing the family's ability to serve as a resource for the patient can have an impact on the decision whether to hospitalize or to treat in an out-patient setting. In most instances, families of suicidal people, like families of cancer patients and heart patients, feel less helpless if they can help with their relative's recovery. They can easily become an important link in the treatment chain.

However, there are times when the family unit is so depleted that they are not a good resource for the client. This is especially true in cases of substance abuse, chronic mental illness or bereavement after the death of a significant family member. In these instances, it may be better to hospitalize the suicidal patient and include intensive family therapy as part of the treatment plan. For example, the team decided to hospitalize a 50-year-old woman with severe suicidal depression when her alcoholic husband refused to participate in the treatment and he was reported to be verbally and physically abusive. The home environment was deemed to be unsafe and unlikely to protect her against her self-destructive impulses.

Culture

Understanding the family's cultural attitudes is crucial in therapeutic intervention. Attitudes about mental illness vary widely across cultures and generations. If the family is to be a part of a treatment plan that decreases the risk of suicide, it is important that these attitudes should be known and factored into the plan. In one of our families, the father was sympathetic to the need for his suicidal son to receive psychiatric treatment. The mother, however, came from a family background that held that problems should be kept within and solved by the family. The clinician learned that he could not count on her to follow through with suggestions that might keep her son safe and so had to rely on the father. Such attitudes are not uncommon and can place the patient in peril if the clinician simply assumes that everyone is in agreement as to the need for treatment.

Suicide in the family

A completed suicide in a family is a devastating event for all surviving family members. They desperately seek an explanation of what has happened. These explanations may run the gamut from denying the cause of the death or attributing it to an accident or murder to blaming other family members for failing the deceased person. Since not everyone in the family is likely to agree with or share the beliefs of everyone else, the family becomes vulnerable to disruption at precisely the time when it is most needed to serve as a source of support for its members. It is widely believed that the earlier the intervention in this instance the better will be the outcome.

In fact, the mental health system as a whole has witnessed a shift in the manner in which survivors of suicides are approached. In the past they were only infrequently contacted (except perhaps to participate in an 'incident review' if the death had occurred while the person was under the care of a psychiatric agency). The folly of this 'hands off' policy is brought home by the fact that people who die by suicide are significantly more likely than others to have been survivors of a loved one's suicide themselves.[5] Regardless of whether this increased risk of suicide among survivors is due to environmental issues or to genetic factors (most probably both elements are at work), it is a situation that calls out for intervention.

Surviving therapist

There are two circumstances in which practitioners may come into contact with survivors, and each requires a different approach. In the first circumstance, the practitioner is the person who has been providing treatment to the victim of suicide. This circumstance creates a period of intense involvement with many different people, some of whom may have goals that are opposite to those of the therapist. Depending on the circumstances, the therapist may be unable to avoid these contacts and can often emerge from the experience feeling blamed by superiors and colleagues and devalued as a clinician. Legal authorities, insurance companies and quality assurance departments may all demand an account from the therapist, seeking to explain this multidetermined event in the simplest terms possible. Frequently, surviving families who know of the clinician's involvement with their loved one will seek an interview in service of their search for explanations about the death. Of course, if the clinician has been involved with the family during the presuicide crisis, the path to the clinician has already been established and family members are likely to pursue it in search of closure. If, on the other hand, the clinician has kept the family distant, they may feel excluded and seek an interview to determine what happened. It has been demonstrated that it is wisest for the surviving therapist to respond positively to the family's request and to be as open as possible about the final weeks and days of treatment, within the bounds of confidentiality. If the therapist has been adhering to the standards of care for a suicidal patient there is generally little to fear from this interview, and it can be enormously helpful to the family. The therapist must view him or herself as a 'survivor' as well, since the death will evoke many of the same emotions experienced by the family. We encourage the therapist to attend some portion of the funeral services if the family welcomes this. We do not recommend that the clinician perform any further clinical services for the family, however. This is best left to third parties, ideally, people with experience of working with surviving families, to whom the clinician should refer the family.

Family's return to the functioning

The second circumstance arises when the therapist is contacted by some distressed surviving family member after a suicide. If the loss is immediate, we recommend that the clinician should meet the whole family several times to assist them in negotiating their grief and help them remain as resources to each other in this process.[6] Such early intervention is often all that is required to get each family member back on track. If the death is less recent or if the family is not available, working with individual family members can be constructive and usually reverberates back to the family system as a whole in a positive fashion. The goal of both family and individual treatment is a return to functioning at a level comparable to that before the death. This entails the following therapeutic tasks:

• educating about grief;

- demystifying suicide;
- eliminating excessive guilt, shame and blaming; and
- assessing and responding to potential suicide risk in the survivors.

Educating about grief

Most people have little experience of grief but many ideas about it, and are therefore surprised when their grieving does not follow a predetermined pattern. This is especially significant for survivors of suicide since they believe that the suicide death itself is disrupting a 'normal' grief process. It is helpful to explore what the survivor's expectations about the process are and to correct any unrealistic expectations that they might have (e.g. 'I'll be over this in a year', or 'I should feel better every day'). We also encourage people to grieve at their own pace while respecting the pace of others. This is particularly salient in a family in which a suicide has occurred, since the family is hypersensitive to the appearance of 'abnormality' and may not be tolerant of other family members' patterns of grieving if they are different from their own.

Demystifying suicide

A suicide is an overdetermined event, although most people seek simple and single explanations for it. It is important that surviving family members broaden their understanding of the factors that led to their loved one's death to include not only disappointment and despair, but also mental illnesses (90 per cent of completed suicide victims can be diagnosed with a major brain-based mental illness) that may have clouded judgment or impaired thinking. The clinician who works with surviving family members should have a deep knowledge base about suicide and should be able to communicate this to the family in terms that they can understand.

Eliminating excessive guilt, shame, and blaming

It is difficult not to place responsibility for a suicide on people other than the victim. Because the victim is not available to explain what happened, suicide heightens the tendency to view either the self or others as more powerful in the situation than they actually were. Exaggerating responsibility can lead to morbid grieving and an unwillingness to forgive the self or disruption in family functioning. The clinician should help survivors achieve a realistic assessment of their role in the situation without undermining their trust in themselves or others.

Assessing and responding to potential suicidal risk in the survivors

The suicide of a loved one plants an idea in the minds of the survivors that somehow suicide is an acceptable solution to life's difficulties. This dangerous idea is what places survivors at increased risk for ending their own life. The clinician should address this issue forthrightly, asking about such thoughts and, while normalizing this as a 'typical' survivor response, helping the survivor to understand the source of the idea. Emphasis must be placed on providing the survivor with the tools and resources needed to overcome such thoughts.

One of the most profound changes in the treatment of survivors of suicide in the past few years has been the development and evolution of support groups. Many different kinds of group exist, with varying degrees of efficacy. What they have in common, however, and what is most useful to survivors, is the presence of others who have undergone a similar experience. These groups deal with the aftermath of suicide compassionately and efficiently. Where available they are really the treatment of choice for survivors. Clinicians should, at the very least, know where such groups are, and help to start them if none exists in the local area.[7]

Case history

Karen, one of the authors of this chapter, received a call from a distraught widower whose wife had just taken her life by using carbon monoxide in her car in a deserted wooded area several miles from their home. She had been in treatment for depression and she seemed to be improving, so her suicide was a shock. She left a note saying that she loved them all but could no longer stand living continually in a numbed state. Her husband was calling for help because he was in conflict with his wife's family about what to tell his children about his wife's death. He wanted to tell them the truth, but his wife's family thought that they should be protected from the knowledge that the death was a suicide.

I explained to him that I felt quite strongly that he should provide the children with the facts, but that he should couple the truth with an explanation of depression and how, when depressed, one's thinking becomes unclear. My conviction comes from 15 years of experience of working with adults who, as children, were not told the truth when their parent died by suicide. Most of the time they were told the death was caused by a heart attack or a car accident, and only found out the real cause of death much later. One survivor told me how he had come to distrust the story he was told. 'Every time they talked about my mother I could hear a catch in their voices. It was like the words not matching the music.' This subsequent discovery of the truth proved to be extremely painful. Survivors frequently describe having to grieve anew each time they learn more information. I suggested to the widower that I would meet with his wife's family and help them understand how important it would be to tell the children the truth.

The meeting went well. The family chose to tell the children that their mother died of a 'brain attack'; that is, the depression clouded her thinking and she was unable to see any other way to solve her problem, likening suicide to a heart attack in which one's heart fails to function properly. I also suggested that the children play a small part in the burial ritual. They were pleased to play a role, and chose pink roses for the church ceremony.

In the months that followed, the widower attended a support group, meeting others with similar experiences. The children attended a weekly group with other bereaved children. Subsequently, the widower told me that some of his closest friends are the parents of the other children in the support group.

In the intervening five years, he remarried and his children, who at times have been in individual therapy to help them through trouble spots, are doing well socially and academically. Each year at the anniversary of their mother's death, they bring pink roses to their church in her memory.

References

1. Alvarez A. A savage God: a study of suicide. New York: Random House; 1970.

2. Shea SC. The practical art of suicide assessment: a guide for mental health professionals and substance abuse counselors. New York: John Wiley and Sons; 1999.

3. McFarlane WR, Dushay R, Lukens E, et al. Multiple family groups in psychoeducational treatment of schizophrenia. *Arch Gen Psychiatry* 1995;**52:**679–687.

4. Jamison KR. Night falls fast: understand suicide. New York: Alfred A Knopf; 1999.

5. Dunne EJ, McIntosh JL, Dunne-Maxim K. Suicide and its aftermath: understanding and counseling the survivors. New York: WW Norton; 1987.

6. Dunne EJ. Psychoeducational intervention strategies for survivors of suicide. *Crisis* 1992; **13:**35–40.

7. World Health Organization. How to start a group of survivors of suicide and be successful. A resource for setting up a self-help support group for those bereaved by suicide. Geneva: World Health Organization; 2000.

VIIB
Public health perspective

29

Perestroika in the former USSR: history's most effective suicide-preventive programme for men

Danuta Wasserman and Airi Värnik

Perestroika: reduced alcohol consumption and a hopeful social climate

Suicide was a prohibited topic in the USSR. Nonetheless, with the major political changes associated with *perestroika* (restructuring) during the Gorbachev regime in the second half of the 1980s, the national archives were opened in 1989. These thus became available for research, making it possible to study, for example, how factors in society at large influence suicide rates. *Perestroika* was characterized by openness and freedom, as well as reform policies. Strict limits were imposed on the sale of alcohol, and a new restrictive attitude towards alcohol consumption was actively encouraged.[1]

Suicides decreased

By using previously classified material about suicide, violent death and alcohol poisoning, we studied statistics on causes of death relating to the whole population in the 15 Soviet Socialist Republics for the years 1970–1990 and various age groups for the years 1984–1990. The highest numbers of suicides were noted in the Slav republics (Russia, Ukraine, Belorussia), Kazakhstan (with its high proportion of Slavs in the population) and the Baltic states (Lithuania, Latvia and Estonia). In these areas the suicide rates were roughly 10 times as high as in the Caucasian states (Armenia, Azerbaijan and Georgia), where the lowest figures were reported. These wide regional variations were largely due to national and cultural differences.[2]

The year 1984 was the last of the period of stagnation (as it may be called) which was characterized by centralization of political and economic power, censorship and isolation from other countries. In 1986–1988, *perestroika* was at a peak. The number of suicides for men in the USSR decreased by 40 per cent in the years 1984–1986 (Figure 29.1), against 3 per cent in 22 European countries studied during the same period. This decline occurred in all 15 republics of the USSR. The largest falls were observed in Russia and Belorussia, where male suicides fell by 42 per cent.[3]

The sharp decrease in suicides applied to women as well as men,[4] but of all groups in the population the largest decrease was among men in the workforce aged between 25 and 54 years – possibly the age range during which one is most responsive to social changes as well as to alcohol policy.[5] No corresponding decline for this age group was noted in any country in the 20th century.[1,6]

These results illustrate history's most effective suicide preventive programme for men. There is no doubt that the sudden decline in suicide rates coincided with the reform period in the USSR known as *perestroika*. It is impossible to state with certainty whether it was hope of a better future, greater freedom or the strict alcohol policy introduced by Gorbachev that brought about the reduction in mortality from violent causes and from stress-related illnesses such as cardiovascular diseases. Both factors were probably important.

These reductions in mortality are not due to statistical errors. Another research group has, like ourselves, shown that the reliability of mortality data was high, and no changes took place in the routines or quality of data collection during *perestroika* compared with the preceding period.[7]

Suicide rates increase when alcohol restriction ends

Unfortunately, the suicide-preventive effects observed during Gorbachev's reforms were not lasting. Unofficial alcohol production rose strikingly after 1988. Scarcity of funds ruled out a continued antialcohol campaign and efforts to change attitudes in the former USSR. Since 1990, there has once more been an explosive rise in suicide rates as well as in overall mortality.[8]

Alcohol restrictions reduce suicides

Several 'natural experiments' – such as Prohibition in the USA in 1910–1920, sharply raised alcohol prices in Denmark in 1911–1924 and restrictions on the sale of alcohol in Sweden in connection with the introduction of ration books in the 1950s – have been proved to cause significant falls in suicide.[9–11]

From clinical studies of suicidal people, it is well known that a sense of hopelessness is a factor that contributes strongly to suicidal thoughts or

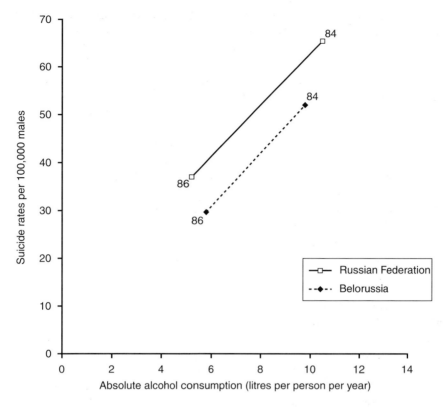

Figure 29.1

Annual suicide rates per 100,000 males and consumption of absolute alcohol in litres per capita in Russian Federation and Belorussia, 1984 and 1986.

acts, and also that alcoholism is an important diagnosis (see Chapter 5). In the light of these facts, the outcome of the vast natural experiment of *perestroika* – that both higher hopes and lower alcohol consumption in the former USSR helped to bring about the most effective suicide-prevention programme for men in our time – are, perhaps, not surprising. Gorbachev's reforms consisted of a combination of various measures, including radical alcohol restrictions, intensive efforts to change attitudes at all levels (from the nation's top political leaders to the 'grass-roots' level) and the introduction of legal sanctions when the basic intentions of the reform were not observed. Production as well as sale of alcoholic beverages fell sharply, owing to governmental restrictions. Compliance with the law at different levels was ensured both by the imposition of various penalties for drunkenness in public or at the workplace, for example, and through effective steps to change attitudes towards the use of alcohol. At every level of Soviet society during the Gorbachev era, for example, proposing toasts in alcohol during official dinners was prohibited. Drinking no longer appeared to be an admired way of asserting one's masculinity.

Alcohol restrictions have different effects in different countries

One may wonder whether alcohol restrictions would have the same impact in other countries with different cultures. Correlations at aggregate level between alcohol consumption and suicide mortality vary from one country to another;[12] thus, the same clear associations between reduced or increased alcohol consumption and correspondingly reduced or increased suicide mortality cannot be discerned in certain countries. Obviously, it is not only the availability of alcohol but how far a society tolerates alcohol and acceptance of alcohol use and abuse that has an impact on the number of alcoholics in the society concerned. In cultures with greater acceptance of alcohol, there are more alcoholics; accordingly, these cultures promote certain forms of behaviour. It is therefore important to understand why, in any particular nation, people drink alcohol.

Alcohol restrictions reduce suicides among alcoholics

Analyses at aggregate level are marred by great uncertainty regarding causality and connections. But a study from Denmark has shown that suicide rates among alcoholics fell when their alcohol consumption decreased as a result of sharp price rises, while the suicide rates among non-alcoholics did not change.[10,13] Studies at the individual level also clearly show the role of alcohol in mortality from suicide and provide additional arguments for interpreting results concerning reductions in suicide during *perestroika*.

Treatment of psychiatric disorders should accompany diminished access to alcohol

However, when measures of suicide prevention are planned, factors other than mere restrictions on the supply of alcohol must be taken into consideration. Suicides among alcoholics are due to a range of psychiatric and psychosocial factors that cannot be influenced solely by reduced access to alcohol. Suicide-prevention measures must therefore include treatment of underlying psychiatric morbidity, reinforcement of social networks and learning of adequate coping strategies to deal with difficult situations, alongside public health measures to regulate access to alcohol.

References

1. Wasserman D, Värnik A, Dankowicz M, Eklund G. Suicide-preventive effects of perestroika in the former USSR: the role of alcohol restriction. *Acta Psychiatr Scand Suppl* 1998;**394:**1–44.

2. Wasserman D, Värnik A, Dankowicz M. Regional differences in the distribution of suicide in the former Soviet Union during perestroika, 1984–1990. *Acta Psychiatr Scand* 1998;**suppl 394:**5–12.

3. Wasserman D, Värnik A, Eklund G. Male suicides and alcohol consumption in the former USSR. *Acta Psychiatr Scand* 1994;**89:** 306–313.

4. Wasserman D, Värnik A, Eklund G. Female suicides and alcohol consumption during perestroika in the former USSR. *Acta Psychiatr Scand* 1998;**suppl 394:** 26–33.

5. Värnik A, Wasserman D, Dankowicz M, Eklund G. Age-specific suicide rates in the Slavic and Baltic regions of the former USSR during perestroika, in comparison with 22 European countries. *Acta Psychiatr Scand* 1998;**suppl 394:**20–25.

6. Wasserman D, Dankowicz M, Värnik A, Olsson L. Suicide trends in Europe, 1984–1990. In: Stefanis CN (ed.). Biopsychosocial approaches to suicide. The Netherlands: Elsevier Science. 1997.

7. Leon D, Chenet L, Shkolnikov V, et al. Huge variation in Russian mortality rates 1984–1994: artefact, alcohol or what? *Lancet* 1997;**350:**383–388.

8. Värnik A. Suicide in the Baltic countries and in the former republics of the USSR. Karolinska Institute, Stockholm: Doctoral dissertation; 1997:1–169.

9. Norström T. Alcohol and suicide in Scandinavia. *Br J Addict* 1988;**83:**553–559.

10. Skog OJ. Alcohol and suicide in Denmark 1911–1924: experiences from a 'natural experiment'. *Addiction* 1993;**88:**1189–1193.

11. Wasserman IM. The impact of epidemic, war, prohibition and media on suicide: United States, 1910–1920. *Suicide Life Threat Behav* 1992;**22:**240–254.

12. Lester D. The association between alcohol consumption and suicide and homicide rates: a study of 13 nations. *Alcohol Alcohol* 1995;**30:**465–468.

13. Skog OJ. Alcohol and suicide: Durkheim revisited. *Acta Sociol* 1991;**34:**193–206.

30
Controlling the environment to prevent suicide

Antoon Leenaars

The main two traditional solutions for preventing suicide in the 20th century have been clinical treatment of suicidal people (i.e. medication, psychotherapy and hospitalization) and the establishment of suicide prevention centres and community programs (e.g. schools). However, there is a third approach to suicide prevention – one of the oldest methods of prevention – which is known as controlling the environment. Removing the sword from the defeated soldier in battle, for example, is an ancient act of prevention. Yet, this prevention tactic has been infrequently discussed until recently. Presumably because most of the work with regard to the prevention and intervention of suicidal behaviour has remained within the realm of clinical settings, this neglect may be understandable, although given current research, too limiting.

Stengel[1] was one of the first to propose controlling the environment as a means for decreasing the incidence of suicide. He noted for example, that the detoxification of domestic gas (from coal gas with high carbon monoxide content to natural gas) might have reduced the suicide rate in nations where the switch had taken place. Subsequent research on the detoxification of domestic gas in England and Wales supported Stengel's proposal. More recently, a review of the research by Clarke and Lester[2] and an international examination by Leenaars et al.[3] from 12 nations validated this approach in treatment.

This perspective on prevention is described in one of the reports of the World Health Organization (WHO) on suicide prevention.[4] Controlling the environment through gun possession control, detoxification of domestic gas, detoxification of car emission, control of availability of the toxic substances, including pharmaceutical drugs, and toning down reports in the press showed clear suicidal preventive effects. They also offered further measures under the rubric of 'other measures'. These too are consistent with environmental approaches, such as fencing high buildings and bridges. There is no definitive evidence for the effectiveness of the 'other measures', but the research, although not 100 per cent conclusive, strongly supports the five measures described below that call for controlling the environment as effective means of reducing suicide.

Gun control

Gun control is often cited as the prototypical example of controlling the environment to prevent suicide. An opportunity for studying the effects of legislative means restriction (e.g. gun control laws) on the use of guns for suicide is provided by Canada's Criminal Law Amendment Act of 1977 (Bill C-51), enforced since 1978. Early commentators on the impact of this Act found little impact on firearm suicide in Canada, but presented only simple charts, with no statistical analysis of the trends. Leenaars and Lester[5] remedied this omission and reported a comprehensive study on the preventive effect on suicide of the Act in Canada. Their study showed that strict firearm control laws suggest that the passage of Bill C-51 may have reduced the use of firearms for suicide. Furthermore, people did not switch to other methods of suicide. Subsequently, Leenaars and Lester showed that the gun control law was most effective with younger people (and least successful with people aged over 65 years) and women. Results on related phenomena on homicide and accidental deaths hold equal promise.

Control of other means of suicide

The tactic of controlling the environment is, however, more complex than gun control, although it is a prototypical example. Referring to gun control as a means for suicide prevention in Canada and in the USA probably makes sense because it is the main method of suicide in these countries. However, in other countries, guns are not a frequent means of suicide. For example, in Cuba, firearms are the least frequent means for committing suicide. In China, pesticides are used very often as a mean of suicide by women living in the rural areas. In other developing countries poisonings with agricultural chemicals are also the most common methods of suicide. The popularity of different suicide methods changes over time and is determined not only by cultural acceptability but also by availability. Thus, one can see great variation in means and, although gun control may make little sense in some regions, the tactic of controlling the environment may still have applicability, as suggested in the WHO report.

Media reporting

Controlling the environment goes beyond issues of the means of suicide. The WHO noted, for example, that there was strong support in research for toning down reports in the press. Several suicidological reports have indicated that there is an association between media reporting about suicides and suicidal behaviour in a society. In Vienna, for example, after the opening of the underground railway system in 1978, it became a common means of suicide. Mass media reported these events in dramatic ways. Subsequently, efforts were made by Etzersdorfer and Sonneck[6] to provide guidelines for media to report suicides. Reports in the media changed and the number of suicides and suicide attempts in the underground railway system dropped by more than 80 per cent and has remained at low levels ever since. Thus, once more, the principle of controlling the environment – in this case media reporting – appears to be useful.

Availability of medications

Controlling the environment is, in fact, not foreign to practicing psychiatrists. Controlling the availability of medications is a common practice, and one of the five steps found to be effective in the prevention of suicide by the WHO. In 1972, Oliver and Hetzel[7] first called attention to the adverse effects of availability of medication. There are variations in mortality rates associated with overdoses of medicines (e.g. antidepressants and sedatives). Common practice calls for prescribed medications to be safe or provided in small amounts to high-risk patients. According to the WHO, this action is consistent with controlling the environment to prevent suicide. The WHO even suggested that the pharmaceutical industry can contribute by providing appropriate dosage units and packages.

Public health action

The approach of controlling the environment is much broader than control of the availability of toxic substances. Examining steps such as gun control and fencing bridges may broaden the understanding of the complex solutions needed to prevent suicide. Not only may this approach have an impact on direct service, but it may also occasion reflection on support of public health action. The detoxification of domestic gas, for example, was supported by the medical research of Kreitman[8] and it has been estimated to have saved uncountable lives. Although further research is needed, restricting access to the tools which aid suicide and the more general approach of controlling the environment may be a viable strategy to prevent suicide in all regions of the world.

Clinical practice

However, despite the recommendations of the WHO and other research, there has been a lack of global impact on clinical practice. The lack of education of patients about means restriction is a clear illustration. The study by Wislar et al.,[9] for example, exemplifies this absence of education. They conducted a chart review of young people receiving mental health evaluation, with 40 per cent being suicide related, in an emergency department of a hospital. Chart reviews provided no evidence that means restriction education was provided. Although further prospective research is needed on the topic, this study and other studies with similar findings call for greater attention to controlling the environment in the treatment of suicidal patients. The lack of education concerning the importance of the restriction of means may be a failure in care, and it applies not only to guns but to other means as well (e.g. the availability of medicines). There are broad global implications of this research in the care and in the failure of care of suicidal persons. Consultations on a difficult case in which there is imminent risk of suicide, especially with lethal means, should be supplemented by protective measures to control environmental factors, such as securing guns and medicines. Therefore, the clinician should not hesitate to ask relevant questions both to the patient and to his or her family.

To conclude, as noted elsewhere in this book, suicide and suicidal behaviors are multifaceted events. This complexity of etiology indicates the necessity of a parallel complexity of solutions. Prevention of suicide and suicidal behaviors can be understood as any action that contributes to decreasing the frequency of the event. The approach known as controlling the environment has been shown to be effective. This third solution to prevention departs from the approaches of traditional treatment and suicide prevention centers and programs; however, in the light of research, this tactic cannot be ignored in clinical practice.

References

1.   Stengel E. Suicide and attempted suicide. Baltimore: Penguin; 1964.

2.   Clarke R, Lester D. Suicide: closing the exits. New York: Springer-Verlag; 1989.

3.   Leenaars A, Cantor C, Connolly J, et al. Controlling the environment to prevent suicide: international perspectives. *Can J Psychiatry* 2000. In press.

4.   Bertolote J, (ed). Guidelines for the primary prevention of mental, neurological and psychosocial disorders: suicide. Geneva: World Health Organization; 1993.

5.   Leenaars A, Lester D. The impact of gun control on suicide: studies from Canada. *Arch Suicide Res* 1998;**4**:25–40.

6.   Etzersdorfer E, Sonneck G. Preventing suicide by influencing

mass-media reporting. The Viennese experience 1980–1996. *Arch Suicide Res* 1998;**4:**67–74.

7. Oliver R, Hetzel B. Rise and fall of suicide rates in Australia: relation to sedative availability. *Med J Aust* 1972;**2:**919–923.

8. Kreitman N. The coal gas story. *Br J Prev Soc Med* 1976;**30:** 86–93.

9. Wislar J, Grossman J, Kruesi J, Fendrich M, Franke C, Ignatowicz N. Youth suicide-related visits in an emergency department serving rural counties: implications for means restriction. *Arch Suicide Res* 1998;**4:**75–87.

31

Suicide clusters and media coverage of suicide

Armin Schmidtke, Sylvia Schaller and Danuta
Wasserman

Suicide clusters

It has long been known that a suicide or suicide attempt may conceivably pave the way for a series – limited in time – of further suicidal acts (attempted suicide and suicide) on the part of susceptible individuals who know the suicide victim, or who hear about the act through mass-media publicity.

Clusters of suicides or suicide attempts may arise, by means of a suggestion effect, among people in the immediate vicinity of the person who attempted or committed suicide[1] – the same school,[2] prison,[3] ward,[4,5] reservation,[6] military unit or as a result of mass-media coverage.[7-13] Cluster suicides and suicide attempts are particularly prevalent among adolescents aged 15–19. An estimated 1–13 percent of all teenage suicides may be categorized as being of the cluster type.[2]

Underlying mechanism

The term 'Werther effect' was coined to describe the phenomenon after the publication of Goethe's *Die Leiden des jungen Werthers* (*The Sorrows of Young Werther*; 1774).[11] In this novel, Werther takes his own life by shooting himself as a result of unrequited love and rejection. Many young people in Europe are believed to have followed Werther's example with the same method and in Italy, Leipzig, Copenhagen and elsewhere the authorities, fearing a wave of juvenile suicides, banned the book.

Identification is a key mechanism in cluster suicides. Susceptible people[1,12] who perceive themselves as helpless and their situation as beyond hope, and who are depressed or otherwise mentally unbalanced can strongly identify with people who have opted to end their lives, unless constructive alternatives are pointed out. An impressionable individual may be influenced by someone else's solution to life's difficulties, and may choose the same self-destructive way out. This is especially true if media reports solely describe the suicide as an inevitable impulsive response to life's stresses and as a glamorous and romantic event, and fail to adequately report the role played by underlying psychiatric illness and psychological problems.

WHO guidelines on media coverage of suicide

There are no controlled studies indicating that a reduction in cluster suicides is attainable through well-designed information inputs. On the other hand, it seems that sensational and irresponsible reporting[9] may contribute to precipitating or inducing suicidal acts. Responsible media coverage can probably counteract suicide contagion and discourage cluster suicides and suicide attempts.[12,14]

WHO has drawn up guidelines on media coverage, prescribing how the press and broadcasting media should report on suicide.[15] It is essential to avoid sensational journalism that describes the suicide victim's attitude as courageous or desirable. There should be no pictures, no detailed descriptions of the suicide method used, nor should the suicide be described as inexplicable, romantic, or as a mysterious act. Psychosocial circumstances that played a part in the decision to die should be elucidated. The role of psychiatric illnesses such as depression, alcohol and substance abuse and the fact that they are treatable must be clarified, and information provided about the care and the help that are available. Positive examples can be presented about how to resolve severe conflicts. The physical consequences of serious suicide attempts, such as brain damage or paralysis, can be described and advice given on how to remedy a difficult life situation and prevent others from committing suicidal acts. Obviously, it is crucial to avoid glorifying, making a martyr of, or creating a mystique around the suicide victim.

The suggestive power of the event can probably be reduced if alternatives to suicide are presented with well-balanced, factual background information about suicidal behaviour and treatment, and also about the scope for prevention. Simultaneously, the names, telephone numbers and addresses of possible sources of assistance should be published.

Prevention of cluster suicidal acts in a psychiatric ward

Cluster suicides or suicide attempts have been described among psychiatric patients having being diagnosed with schizophrenia, major depression, alcohol dependency and histrionic or borderline personality structure. When a suicide or suicide attempt takes place in a psychiatric ward, it is vital to offer support and present positive identification models to all the patients, but especially to the persons at risk in order to reduce the risk of ensuing cluster suicidal acts. People who commit cluster suicidal acts are often already manifest suicidal or thinking about this possibility. Susceptible people and their suicidality is activated through identification with the deceased, or with the act as a solution to life's difficulties if a suicide takes place in their surroundings.

In providing information doctors should – with objectivity and without idealization – show respect for the deceased and grief at the loss, but simultaneously point out that the wish to commit suicide is almost always ambivalent and that this solution is not the most reasonable way to address the problems. An objective description of how to treat the mental illness and cope with the mental and psychosocial stress, and how a suicidal process can be affected, among other factors, by interaction with significant others (see Chapter 2) should be provided. It is vital to engage both the care staff and the other patients on the ward in listing various constructive options for solving problems which probably contributed to their fellow patient's suicide, as well as to emphasise the importance of confiding in the staff about any pressing suicidal thoughts that arise, and of being open to treatment and support. It should also be explained to patients that informing staff of other patients' suicidal intentions is necessary and is not a form of denunciation.

If there is a patient on the ward who has previously attempted suicide or had very pronounced suicidal ideation, regular suicide-risk assessment should be carried out. In addition the treatment provided should be supplemented by intense psychotherapy to work through possible identification with the patient who committed suicide.

References

1. Hazell P. Adolescent suicide clusters: Evidence, mechanisms and prevention. *Australian and New Zealand Journal of Psychiatry* 1993;**27**:653–665.

2. Gould MS. Teenage suicide clusters. JAMA 1990b;**263**:2051–2052.

3. Cox B, Skegg K. Contagious suicide in prisons and police cells. *Journal of Epidemiology and Community Health* 1993;**47:** 69–72.

4. Rissmiller DJ, Rissmiller F. Inpatient suicide epidemics and suggestions for prevention. Hospital and community psychiatry *Hosp Community Psychiatry* 1990;**41:**922–924.

5. Taiminen TJ, Helenius H. Suicide clustering in a psychiatric hospital with a history of a suicide epidemic: A quantitative study. *American Journal of Psychiatry* 1994;**151:**1087–1088.

6. Rubinstein DH. Epidemic suicide among Micronesian adolescents. *Social Science and Medicine* 1983;**17:**657–665.

7. Hankoff LD. An epidemic of attempted suicide. *Comprehensive Psychiatry* 1961;**2:**294–298.

8. Etzersdorfer E, Sonneck G, Nagel-Kuess S. Newspaper reports and

suicide. *N Eng J Med* 1992;**327:** 502–503.

9. Marzuk PM, Tardiff K, Hirsch CS et al. Increase in suicide by asphyxiation in New York City after the publication of Final Exit. *N Engl J Med* 1993;**329(20):** 1508–10.

10. Philips DP, Carstensen LL. Clustering of teenage suicides after television news stories about suicide. *N Eng J Med* 1986;**315:** 685–689.

11. Schmidtke A, Hafner H. The Werther effect after television films: New evidence for an old hypothesis. *Psychological Medicine* 1988;**18:**665–676.

12. Schmidtke A, Schaller S. The role of mass media in suicide prevention. In: K Hawton and K van Heeringen (eds). The International Handbook of Suicide and Attempted Suicide. New York: Wiley. 2000:675-697.

13. Stack S. The effect of the media on suicide: evidence from Japan, 1955-1985. *Suicide Life Threat Behav* 1996;**26(2):**132-42.

14. Berman A, Jobes DA, O'Carroll P. The aftermath of Kurt Cobain's suicide. In De Leo D, Schmidtke A, Diekstra RFW. Suicide Prevention: a Holistic Approach. 1997: 139–143.

15. World Health Organization, Geneva 2000. Preventing suicide: A resource for media professionals. Department of Mental Health, Social Change and Mental Health.

32
Examples of suicide prevention in schools

Danuta Wasserman and Véronique Narboni

Starting suicide prevention early

Conducting suicide prevention among young people is a highly responsible task and one that requires careful consideration.[1,2] The fact that young people are impressionable, open to new ideas and sometimes uncritical is part of their charm. Unfortunately, this juvenile tendency to absorb new impressions uncritically and to be easily influenced by others may sometimes have grave and harmful consequences. Adolescents are influenced by music, fashion and youth idols – not only in terms of clothing and hairstyle, but also in their attitudes towards drugs, alcohol and aspects of behaviour that are both desirable and undesirable.

It is not surprising that both good and bad models find imitators among teenagers. Sadly, suicides and suicide attempts in youth settings are sometimes provoked by incautiously imparted information.[3-5] This happens when young people's fantasies are stimulated by a preoccupation with a notion of suicide that is glorified and sensationalized: they identify with the self-destructive existence of people who have committed suicidal acts, when such a life is portrayed as 'romantic' and attractive.

School as an arena for promotion of mental health and prevention of suicide

Children spend many hours a day at school. The school setting also affords scope for monitoring not only their physical development but also of their cognitive and emotional growth, their emergent sexuality and their social-role adjustment. The education system is a suitable arena for introducing programmes to promote mental health and prevent suicide and for establishing policies and procedures that can be adopted by the whole school system and by people working at individual schools.

Topics relating to mental health and suicide prevention may be naturally woven into the school curriculum, just like teaching about reproduction, sexuality and physical health. Instructions may also be given that not only the pupils, but the school staff and the parents as well, should have the opportunity to take part in tailored educational programmes.

Prevention of mental disorders and psychological distress early in the life cycle is highly important, given the wide-ranging adverse repercussions of mental disorders in terms not only of suicidality, but also of children's and adolescents' scholastic performance and formation of social networks. Giving children and adolescents balanced skills for coping with life requires efforts not only on their parents' part but also from other adults – parents of children's friends, family friends and school staff. This is particularly important when many children in the contemporary world come from broken families or live with parents who are incapable of giving them the support that a growing child needs.

Mental ill-health and suicidal behaviour among school pupils

Depression among young people is becoming more prevalent, and it is occurring at an ever lower age. Many children experience anxiety and stress, both in the family and at school. Several studies have shown that suicidal ideation is common at puberty, but even among children below the age of 12 years, up to 9 per cent have such thoughts.

In a Swedish survey of adolescents aged 15–17 years, up to 8 per cent of girls and 3 per cent of boys self-report that they have attempted suicide. A psychiatric evaluation applying strict criteria for defining attempted suicide shows that 2 per cent of boys and 4 per cent of girls have in fact tried to take their own lives. International investigations reveal similar results.[2] These alarming figures show that many young people are experiencing severe distress and that, among school pupils, there is a strikingly large group who would benefit from psychological and psychiatric measures of an interventional or postventional nature and who require intensive and skilled psychological, psychiatric and social input. If this fact is not taken into account in programmes of health promotion and suicide prevention, ill-advised information campaigns may actually trigger suicide attempts or suicides among these already vulnerable young people, instead of preventing them.[5,6]

Among the remainder – the majority of adolescents, who are well and happy – health-promoting or suicide-preventive inputs that are not carefully considered may encounter both indifference and resistance. In some cases, they may arouse curiosity about experimenting with drugs and alcohol or self-destructive behaviour. For this reason, health-promotion and suicide-preventive inputs cannot be left to enthusiastic amateurs or artists in the world of film, theatre or music. Today, we know that very close co-operation between professionals and artists is needed to reach young people both intellectually and emotionally and to stimulate them to mature and develop balanced lifestyles of their own choice.

Knowledge and attitudes can be influenced

The fact that psychoeducative programmes enhance awareness and boost knowledge of mental health and suicidal behaviour has been documented. A small number of studies have focused on changes in attitudes. Esters et al.[7] describe significant and sustained improvement in attitudes towards seeking psychiatric treatment, in a programme that emphasized educating pupils about mental illness and the roles of various mental-health professionals. But can suicidal behaviour be reduced? We know from scientific reports that ill-considered information can boost it. But it is plausible to assume that young people's development can also be influenced in a positive direction, by giving them a chance to identify with, and emulate, good models.

Behaviour can be influenced

As yet, there have been few studies to show that programmes of suicide prevention and intervention can change suicidal behaviour (i.e. reduce the numbers of suicides and attempted suicides). One of the best implemented and scientifically documented studies has been a 5-year study of suicidal behaviour among school pupils who participated in a prevention and intervention programme in Dade County Public Schools (DCPS), Miami, Florida, USA.[8] In this ambitious and well-designed programme (described briefly below) it was possible, using intervention inputs, to reduce the number of suicides by 62 per cent and the number of suicide attempts from 87 to 31 per 100,000. A significant reduction in suicide attempts after a brief prevention and intervention programme in Stockholm schools has also been demonstrated.

Policy-creating suicide-preventive programmes and broad support

Zenere and Lazarus[8] documented a comprehensive, district-wide Suicide Prevention and School Crisis Management Program of several years' duration in DCPS. The programme was based on a threefold approach – prevention, intervention and postvention – adapted for a total of some 330,000 pupils at the state's elementary, middle and senior high schools. For the youngest pupils, the teaching was arranged in such a way that they developed their self-awareness and communication skills, learned to make decisions and were given models of positive alternative ways of resolving various conflicts. They were also taught to find alternatives to abuse of alcohol and drugs, to develop their relationships, to perceive ways of dealing with stress and to resist group pressure.

For older pupils, the programme had greater depth. They learned, for example, about conflict resolution, decision-making, stress management and so forth. The pupils also had a chance to learn about psychological defence mechanisms, making their own active choices and becoming aware of factors that affect health and well-being. Knowledge of how and where to seek help was also provided.

The educational programme was implemented by trained and specially selected teachers and mental-health professionals. All the pupils in the DCPS system have undergone this syllabus. Moreover, a school-based crisis team, comprising eight to 10 professionals – social workers, psychologists, school social workers, teachers and other staff – was established at each school. Team members were selected with reference to their occupation, skill and interest in the problem concerned. A scheme had also been devised concerning the ways in which every school and team, at regular intervals, was to be updated in terms of knowledge, programme implementation and collection of research data for evaluation of the programme.

All the parents were informed about the programme and could also attend courses about the problems concerned. School administrative staff received information and supported the policies and the formalized training programme, which were implemented throughout the school workforce. Government and other agencies in the catchment area were also informed. This meticulous preparation and implementation permitted prompt and effective intervention and postvention to help vulnerable children and adolescents, since everyone was prepared to carry out the requisite measures.

At what age should pupils be taught about suicidal behaviour?

In Florida, the choice was made to introduce teaching about juvenile suicide and various strategies for dealing with stress and resolving conflicts in a mandatory one-term syllabus at 10th-grade level (15-year-olds).

In several Stockholm schools, a programme of suicide prevention was first implemented for pupils in the first and second years of upper-secondary school (aged 16–17 years) and later in classes 8 and 9 of primary school (aged 14–15 years). The design of the Stockholm programme corresponds to the Florida programme of life-management skills but is much shorter. The school management and the entire school staff were trained in mental health and ill-health topics and in suicide prevention. The programme was implemented in experimental classes and the results were compared with control classes. The parents were informed of the experiment, as were the health-care authorities in the area.

The programme for Stockholm pupils is composed of lectures on the following 11 themes:

- how emotion influences stress;
- identity development;
- mental crisis;
- stress during the school years;
- bullying;
- depression in the young;
- suicidal thoughts;
- suicide attempts and suicide;
- an integrated approach to health (medical, psychological and social);
- psychosocial working conditions in the classroom; and
- how music, art and poetry can be used in reflection about one's own health.

Brief theoretical lessons were supplemented by psychodrama and role-play exercises in which pupils could act out various conflicts and identify solutions. The programme was implemented by a school nurse and social worker, with support from other health-care professionals and teachers.[9]

The programme was evaluated in terms of skills in communication with peers and adults, and in terms of the number of suicide attempts. The results are described below.

Communication with peers and adults was significantly improved. The confidentiality issue was discussed and the message that seeking professional help for a friend in distress is not betrayal was emphasized. Confidentiality, which young people do not know how to handle, is often the reason why most pupils do not heed the advice they have received about how to deal with a distressed friend.

Moreover, school pupils were given the message that they do not need to be alone with their problems and that they should seek professional help. The main objective was to remove the stigma of guilt and shame about psychological distress and psychiatric disorders, and to liken it to somatic illness. To promote help-seeking behaviour, pupils were given leaflets about the resources available in the community and how to make use of traditional case-management procedures.

There was a decrease in attempted suicide in the experimental group compared with a control group. However, more trials are required to confirm the positive results from suicide-preventive activities in the USA and Sweden.

Suicide attempts and suicides among adolescents can be prevented

The results of both the above-mentioned studies show that the numbers of suicides and suicide attempts can be significantly reduced. In other words, behaviour can be modified. Nonetheless, suicidal thoughts – possibly an indicator of psychological make-up and defence mechanisms – was unchanged. Accordingly, with psychoeducative and cognitive methods, behaviour can be modified: young people can be induced to seek help in difficult situations and to choose solutions other than suicide attempts and suicide when problems arise.

Suicide prevention among pupils is not necessarily controversial

It is important to implement suicide-preventive measures in schools rigorously, carefully and with great awareness. This is because there is a great danger of precipitating, instead of preventing, suicidal acts if such programmes are run by unprofessional people with a leaning towards the dramatic aspects of the subject and a craving for sensation. Psychoeducational programmes targeted on pupils sometimes use videotaped accounts by teenagers of their own suicide attempts, or stage drama. It is important to be sure how characters in the films or plays are perceived by pupils involved in the preventive programme. The adverse experience from various short-lived information or educational campaigns has taught us a lesson. The lesson is that suicide-prevention measures must be implemented in conjunction with measures to promote health and prevent mental ill-health, on a long-term basis and in a carefully considered way.[1,2]

Co-operation with health-care professionals

Suicide prevention in schools must be conducted in close collaboration with psychiatrists, psychologists and other professionals in order to support pupils, their parents and the school staff in dealing with suicidal adolescents. Co-operation with community organizations, local authorities and health agencies, churches and voluntary organizations is a prerequisite for success.

Co-operation with parents

It is, moreover, important to remember that management of children and adolescents in distress and at risk of suicide should be carried out by a team in intimate co-operation with the pupils' parents and families.

School staff's work environment

Strengthening the mental health of school staff is also of the utmost importance. Teachers are in charge of young people who represent the future of every nation. For teachers and other staff, the workplace can be hostile, with aggression and sometimes even violence. School staff therefore need information material that enhances their understanding and proposes adequate reactions to mental strain and mental illness among their colleagues and pupils. They should also have access to support and, if necessary, treatment.

References

1. Shaffer D, Gould M. Suicide prevention in schools. In: Hawton K, van Heeringen K (eds). Suicide and attempted suicide. John Wiley and Sons; 1999:645–660.

2. Wasserman D, Narboni V. Preventing suicide: a resource for school teachers and other school staff. World Health Organization. Geneva. 2000.

3. Phillips DP, Carstensen LL. Clustering of teenage suicides after television news stories about suicide. *N Engl J Med* 1986; **315:**685–689.

4. Schmidtke A, Häfner H. The Werther effect after television films: new evidence for an old hypothesis. *Psychol Med* 1988;**18:**665–676.

5. Schmidtke A, Schaller S. What do we do about media effects on imitation of suicidal behaviour. In: De Leo D, Schmidtke A, Schaller S (eds). Suicide prevention: a holistic approach. Dordrecht, The Netherlands: Kluwer Academic Publishers; 1998:121–137.

6. Hazell P. Adolescent suicide clusters: evidence, mechanisms and prevention. *Aust N Z J Psychiatry* 1993;**27:**653–665.

7. Esters IG, Cooker PG, Ittenbach RF. Effects of a unit of instruction in mental health on rural adolescents' conceptions of mental illness and attitudes about seeking help. *Adolescence* 1998;**33:** 469–476.

8. Zenere FJ, Lazarus PJ. The decline of youth suicidal behavior in an urban, multicultural public school system following the introduction of a suicide prevention and intervention program. *Suicide Life Threat Behav* 1997;**27:**387–402.

9. Ahlner B, Hildingsdotter Bengtsson E. Mentally preventive healthcare – a teaching material in life competence. Täby: Sama förlag AB; 1996.

Index